Awake all Hours

The story of the New Zealand junior doctors' rebellion of 1985.

Dr Jeremy Cooper with Selwyn Parker

Awake all Hours

Table of Contents

Chapter one

Terrifying responsibilities

A junior doctor had been on duty for nearly 72 hours. In all that time he had been able to snatch only a few hours sleep and now he was helping operate on a patient with fractures while fighting to stay awake. The patient's leg had been opened up and the specialist was conducting a careful procedure as the junior doctor held back the edges of the wound with a retractor.

Suddenly, he began to feel faint and his head tipped towards the surgical area. Just before he collapsed into the open wound, the specialist moved quickly and elbowed him out of the way. "Go home and rest," he ordered. "You're hindering the surgery, not helping it." Chastened, the junior doctor did as he was told, knowing that he could have compromised the sterility of the wound and caused serious harm to the patient. He went off to the doctors' residence and snatched a few hours sleep before returning to duty.

This incident occurred in the early 1980s in New Zealand, a time when junior doctors in hospitals in New Zealand, Britain, USA and much of the western world were expected to work extreme hours that had been banned by law in other occupations for decades. Yet somehow the practice of requiring some of the most talented, highly trained and dedicated people to put in shifts that brought them to the brink of emotional and physical collapse remained firmly entrenched in thousands of hospitals.

This had occurred despite an existing -- and growing -- body of research that identified the consequences of such prolonged periods of sleeplessness. For instance, the emotional toll taken by the *content* of virtually endless hours on the wards rather than their mere *number* was severe. Not only were junior doctors reeling from physical exhaustion, they were often crushed by the emotional fatigue resulting from the gravity of their responsibilities. According to the numerous studies on the subject, then and now, it typically takes longer to recover from emotional exhaustion than it does from physical fatigue, which was why these trainee doctors suffered an alarming and disproportionate number of crashes when they drove themselves home, their hand and eye coordination having declined sharply. As researchers had already identified, their condition was similar to drunk drivers.

But the emotional toll was perhaps the gravest consequence. In the United States, for example, there was unequivocal evidence that suicide rates among junior doctors ("residents" in America) stood at three to eight times those applying in other sectors of employment. The use of alcohol and drugs was unusually high. Divorce rates were off the scale. As Time magazine would soon write in an investigation of the situation: "The hours are endless. The pay is paltry. The tasks are often menial. The responsibilities are terrifying."

Since the 1980s one study after another has continued to confirm these conclusions while also raising another issue of vital importance in acute medicine. Namely, that the functionality of seriously sleep-deprived people becomes increasingly impaired the longer they stay on their feet, however well trained they may be. This is of course precisely why the operational hours of airline pilots, nuclear power workers, long-distance truck drivers and other members of the working population whose efficient performance is fundamental to the safety of the wider public have long been strictly regulated by law, with serious legal consequences for any breaches.

Just one example of the substantial library of research on the subject, a study by the British Columbia Medical Journal has identified specific categories of impairment in ability that result from – or are associated with -- lack of sleep or broken sleep. One of these was defined as "performance nadir", the state in which people find themselves when attempting to work effectively between 3am-5am. Another category was "sleep inertia", a condition that means severely rest-deprived individuals are likely to perform well below their full capacity, whatever the time of day, but particularly so when they are woken from a deep sleep. As the journal pointed out, this is often the time when junior doctors are immediately required to perform at a high level because of an emergency.

As the researchers put it: "Cognitive performance is typically sub-maximal immediately upon awakening because of [this] phenomenon. Sleep inertia's effects are most apparent during the initial 10 to 15 minutes after awakening, but they may take hours to dissipate."

Obviously, any sharp decline in "cognitive performance" is of concern to an individual who is engaged in a task that requires their full capacities, but it is surely more so for those in critical occupations.

As the journal concluded: "The impact of sleep inertia is particularly relevant to residents since they are frequently required to complete complex processes immediately after waking at night. Patient assessment involves a significant degree of evaluative thinking and often necessitates quick, high-impact decision making. A physician must accurately order medications and tests and may be called upon to quickly perform invasive procedures that require considerable concentration and skill. The cognitive impairment attributed to sleep inertia negatively affects the ability to complete these tasks and poses a serious barrier to effective care."

The study went on to show that surgical residents who had been awake the previous night made 20 percent more errors and took 14 percent longer when conducting laparoscopic procedures (popularly known as "keyhole" surgery) than those who arrived fresh on the ward.

Nearly all junior doctors could cite experiences that proved exactly these conclusions. One New Zealand doctor, who had been toiling an epic 80-hour stint that had started at 8am on Friday and would not end until 5pm at the earliest the following Monday, recalls that he was so exhausted by the Monday afternoon that he was unable to perform one of the simplest of procedures – inserting a cannula that introduces intravenous fluids. In short, a drip.

If anything, the early findings about slumps in performance by sleep-deprived doctors have proved to be conservative. Subsequent studies have established that the surgical error rate of chronically fatigued doctors could be as high as 35.9 percent while the percentage of serious diagnostic errors rose by 5.6 times, meaning that patients might easily be undergoing treatment for the wrong condition. Before and since, all the evidence has established beyond reasonable doubt that wide-awake doctors do a better job than half-asleep ones.

Health and emotional considerations aside, such marathon periods of work meant that lower-ranking doctors had no time for a normal life in the accepted sense. Given there are 168 hours in every seven days, the 90-hour week that many of them spent in the hospitals in the eighties and earlier left exactly 56 non-working hours. If they could manage an average six hours a night sleep, which was by no means guaranteed, that left two hours a day for everything else including eating, relaxing, exercising and, of course, the studying that was an essential component of further training. It was a tribute to the commitment of junior doctors that surprisingly few cracked under the strain, an achievement they often attribute to a mutually supportive team that pulled each other through the darkest times.

But why had such an indefensible situation been allowed to develop in western hospitals?

The method of training up junior doctors was seen almost as a baptism of fire, a tradition that had arisen for a variety of seemingly good reasons. In their day most of the senior medical hierarchy had undergone a similar medical boot camp and they saw it as an apprenticeship that produced the best doctors. Extreme tiredness, it was said, came with the territory. It had become a kind of mantra. As junior doctors in New Zealand were routinely told: "You've got to learn to practise medicine when fatigued because you're going to have to work when exhausted all your lives."

Trainees got much the same message elsewhere around the world, and certainly in the United States. "For decades doctors have argued the merits of medical residency – the gruelling and sleepless years of specialty training that constitute a rite of passage into medical practice in America," Time magazine wrote. "Senior physicians defend the traditional residency as a necessary part of the toughening-up process for professionals who must deal with emergencies and late-night awakenings throughout their careers."

The prevailing assumption in hospitals, you might say, was that trainee doctors had to learn to suffer.

But this wasn't just about standing on your feet until you dropped. It was considered that dealing with many patients, sometimes a hundred or more in a single shift in a busy acute ward, was the most effective way of learning medicine. In training, it was quantity that counted. Among New Zealand's junior doctors this was sarcastically known as "mileage" -- and the same principle had become holy writ around the world.

There was another argument in support of 90-hour weeks that bore more merit -- it was called continuity-of-care. This held that the first doctor to see a patient should follow through until the individual was considered to be out of danger. This was thought preferable to handing the case over to a relieving doctor who might miss something important in the briefing and inadvertently apply a treatment that was unsuitable or dangerous. Over many decades, the principle of continuity-of-care had become entrenched in hospitals in the acute wards and junior doctors were routinely expected to stay on their feet – or at least be available – for as many hours as was necessary after an emergency operation, particularly if the patient's life hung in the balance. Like most of the other assumptions that lay behind punishingly long hours on the wards, continuity-of-care had never been subjected to thorough and objective analysis.

One obvious question that merited analysis was: how many seriously ill patients would prefer the attention of an exhausted doctor over a fresh one?

The entrenched ideas that underpinned these hours were not entirely the fault of the senior hospital hierarchy -- junior doctors themselves were partly to blame. As members of a highly principled profession, they had absorbed during their six years of study at medical school a compelling sense of responsibility towards the sick. Exhausted though they might be, junior doctors were almost preconditioned not to leave patients in the lurch. As one New Zealand house surgeon told a magazine shortly before the rebellion that is the subject of this book was launched against the system: "You're entitled to refuse [an extra shift after a 75-hour week] but what happens if you do? *Somebody* has to do it. The patients aren't just going to get up and cure themselves. They can't force you to do it, but you do it anyway."

Another, more material, reason why junior doctors took a stoical view of this harsh apprenticeship was the promise of longer-term rewards, the light at the end of a very long tunnel. Although they were doctors in only the most technical sense, having provisional registration for just one year under the New Zealand system, most were ambitious and had their sights set on bigger things. The steps up the medical ladder were clearly defined. If they made the grade in the first year (which was by no means a certainty), they would qualify to become second-year house surgeons with full registration, a position that gave them a more permanent foothold in the system.

At the end of their term of duty as house surgeons they faced an important choice. They could opt for general practice or they could embark on another and perhaps more challenging career path, that of the specialist in a preferred discipline. The latter entailed more years of toil as a junior doctor, albeit increasingly experienced and respected, from which they emerged with the title of registrar. This step up the ladder was a particularly onerous one because registrars were expected to perform all their normal medical duties while educating and guiding the house surgeons under their wing. It also helped if registrars developed advanced diplomatic skills because they acted as a link in the chain that led all the way up to the consultants ("attendings" in America) who occupy the senior positions in most hospitals.

If they continued to make the grade, registrars then faced further intense and advanced training that left little time for any other activities. In New Zealand, that entailed at least four years of study which included notoriously difficult exams. If they were successful in those (many failed and had to re-sit), registrars generally sought a position overseas for another two or more years where they would gain even more experience. After that they could return to New Zealand if they chose to do so and be granted the title of junior consultant – that is, a member of the second-ranking tier in the hospital hierarchy.

Therefore at the end of a long and arduous road, the junior specialist had completed at least eight or more years of training in the system on top of their years in medical school, followed by several more in hospitals in New Zealand or elsewhere. By then, he or she would be in their early thirties, the boot camp of their years as junior doctors having faded to an unpleasant memory. "I hardly remember anything of my twenties," one specialist remembers. "They just went missing."

But in the early eighties there were moves afoot to reform the system. "Who wants to put his life in the hands of a novice who has been on duty for 26 consecutive hours?" Time would ask rhetorically, echoing the conclusion of the body of research that had already appeared.

In America, the more thoughtful physicians were growing concerned at the size of the responsibilities being heaped on inexperienced – and probably exhausted -- shoulders. In the eighties, as we will see, interns and residents in New York commonly worked up to 95 hours a week and non-stop shifts of 24 hours were routine. One of the critics of the system was Dr. Bertrand Bell, an expert in emergency medicine who worked at the Bronx Municipal Health Centre, an institution often overwhelmed by patients suffering from various kinds of trauma. As he would soon argue in an enquiry that made the headlines, far too much was expected of these young doctors who were, after all, only "graduate medical students and (some) fresh out of medical school." Dr. Bell was particularly outspoken about the inadequate supervision they received from more experienced doctors, although this was one of the key principles often cited in support of medical boot camp.

It was in late 1984 that a group of junior doctors in New Zealand decided the situation had become so intolerable that they must do something about it. Little did they know that in the fulness of time they would lead the world in catalysing reforms for junior doctors' working hours that attracted considerable interest in other countries.

The ginger group was fully aware of the heavy odds stacked against them. Apart from in New Zealand, there had been sporadic outbreaks of rebellion in several countries in the previous decade, notably in Britain, certain Scandinavian countries and the United States. None of these campaigns had succeeded in reducing the hours to a level that would be considered reasonable – or lawful -- in other workplaces.

Chapter two

Undertime

The reform-minded junior doctors believed they had identified a rare window of opportunity. New Zealand's long-running National government had just been defeated and replaced by a Labour administration that they hoped might look favourably on their proposals to put a stop to the virtually unlimited hours expected of them.

"It was our best chance of success in many years," remembers Dr Jeremy Cooper, one of the ringleaders. "We believed we could have a real go at the issue. Something had to be done, and workers' rights were a shining issue for the Labour government."

It was Cooper who had nearly collapsed into the open wound during orthopaedic surgery and been packed off to get some sleep, but his determination to change things had been reinforced on many other occasions. He had also shared long discussions with colleagues about junior doctors' conditions and, although their degree of militancy varied, nearly all of them were willing to throw their weight into a campaign and help in whatever way they could.

An inner circle of supporters soon developed, all of them motivated by their individual experiences of mind-numbing fatigue. None of them laboured under any illusions about the size of the challenge ahead of them. As previous history showed all too clearly, this would be a David-and-Goliath encounter.

The last major campaign to improve the lot of junior doctors had occurred ten years earlier. It had been launched in mid-1975 by the Auckland branch with Gordon Howie as president. Another junior doctor, Lloyd Cairns, was secretary of the national association. Then a house surgeon in Auckland Hospital's A&E department, Howie got involved in a battle that became folklore in the health system, in part because of the opposition it aroused among the medical hierarchy.

Howie was motivated by the unfairness of the situation in which he and his colleagues found themselves. They sometimes had to work 56-hour non-stop shifts between 8am

Saturday and 5pm Monday, generally the busiest period in a general hospital during which they routinely dealt with life-and-death cases. They usually did so without the presence of senior doctors and even registrars who, although officially on call, were often reluctant to attend A&E in person.

In the days before acute admitting wards were established, the pressure in A&E was relentless, building up steadily during the Saturday afternoon and reaching a climax around 11.30pm. By then the waiting rooms in A&E were crowded with scores of patients suffering from a wide variety of ailments and injuries. Sports injuries were the most common, and particularly those received in rugby -- a sign over the door read: "Please remove your boots." Other traumas were self-inflicted such as cuts, bruises, broken limbs, concussions and worse that were incurred in drink-fuelled street fights and high-speed car crashes – seat belts were infrequently worn and this was the era before median barriers made roads safer. Other patients arrived with chronic and life-threatening conditions such as asthma. Drug overdoses were common, for instance from barbiturates such as Seconal, and the staff quickly became highly skilled at high-speed stomach wash-outs. Auckland Hospital's proximity to the red-light district around Karangahape Road at the top of the city added to the pressure -- A&E was the first port of call for sex workers. This torrent of patients was rapidly assessed in the admitting wards and, if necessary, passed on to the medical, surgical and psychiatric teams for urgent attention.

It was standard practice to deal with 30 or 40 patients in a weekend but sometimes Howie and his single colleague would treat up to a hundred, hurrying from case to case for hours on end.

The junior doctors had little or no idea what might be coming through the door. On one occasion a young Polynesian woman was brought in as she took almost her last gasp. She was bleeding from what appeared to be a small chest wound. But when staff performed a quick chest drain, it produced a huge volume of blood. By great good luck, a colleague happened to be passing by in the corridor after conducting cardiac surgery. He took one look at the patient and whipped her into theatre where he sewed up the ventricle in the nick of time. Later, the woman, who was single, remorsefully revealed that she had tried to commit suicide by stabbing herself with a steak knife after discovering she was pregnant.

Nearly all junior doctors had their stories of emergency medicine conducted *in extremis*. In the mayhem the one sure ally was the nursing staff -- "they were fabulous, you couldn't have done it without them," Howie recalled 40 years later.

Only once did he and his colleagues get an unexpected respite from the ever-accelerating treadmill of emergency medicine. When the city's brewery workers went on strike and the pubs ran dry, the number of people turning up for treatment with wounds inflicted in fights, or with severe headaches and belly aches, collapsed immediately. On one Saturday night in fact, the A&E department at Auckland Hospital was almost deserted. Although the reason for the abrupt decline in the number of cases did not say much for human behaviour, at least the medical team had a decent weekend's sleep for the first time in months. When the strike ended after nine weeks and the beer started flowing again, normal business was resumed.

The financial rewards for this devotion to duty were meagre, to say the least. Junior doctors were paid for a 40-hour week, however long they worked. Even if they worked more than twice as many hours, which they usually did, they still ended up with the same income because there was no such thing as recompense for overtime. In short, junior doctors including house surgeons and registrars were required to provide for free all work over and above 40 hours a week, as though they were a charity. This meant there was no incentive for management to reduce their hours.

Another sore point for Howie was that junior doctors were excluded from rights that had long been enshrined in industrial law, not only in their home country but in most western nations. Unlike the situation in every other trade and profession, the work rosters of junior doctors did not recognise any public or statutory holidays, such as in the form of compensation through days off or extra earnings.

So, having been elected on a ticket of addressing these injustices, Howie promptly drew up the battle lines. They were based on three principal issues: four weeks annual leave (the same as most people in the New Zealand workforce enjoyed at that period), some form of overtime pay after the first 40 hours, and an absolute maximum of 80 hours a week for any reason (this was twice the average working week).

The obvious implication of Howie's conditions was that hospitals would be forced to hire a bigger pool of junior doctors to plug the manpower gap in the front lines of medicine – and to date they had demonstrated no intention of doing so. The managers of the nation's health system had dug in their heels on this issue for so long – and got away with it – that they were confident the Howie campaign would go the way of all the previous ones.

However when the media got wind of the campaign, the newspapers and television overwhelmingly took the junior doctors' side. "When the largest hospital in the country is unable to find a replacement house surgeon at short notice for night duty in the A&E ward, the staff is clearly stretched beyond reasonable limits," editorialised the New Zealand Herald. The manpower crisis, it went on, was symptomatic of the "hand to mouth" way the city's hospital services were managed.

The issue of excessive hours went deeper than junior doctors' fatigue because it touched directly on quality of patient care, the very principle on which the Hippocratic Oath was based. As a former president of the junior doctors' organisation had explained at the launch of an earlier abortive campaign: "We have been able to give barely satisfactory medical care. [The situation is] hard on the patients, hard on us and hard on our families." It was a plea from the heart, an echo of what the mounting research into the consequences of excessive hours was establishing beyond reasonable doubt.

Howie immediately ran into flak from the medical establishment. "Your career's shot if you carry on like this," one senior doctor told him bluntly. Particularly upset was the senior surgeons committee, a highly influential body. Its viewpoint was not an insignificant consideration for junior doctors. Warnings from the medical hierarchy of the career consequences of any attempt to remedy the junior doctors' conditions had stopped earlier militants dead in their tracks. After all, this was a profession where the establishment held most of the cards. Anybody with ambitions to become a specialist had to be selected by senior specialists for a specific training scheme – obstetrics, for instance -- but competition for the very few places available was so keen that only a handful could be accepted. Up to 40 applicants might apply for the most sought-after schemes, so it was unwise to incur the wrath of the very people who chose the entrants.

Some of the senior doctors, recalling their own trainee years, saw agitation for a limited number of hours as incompatible with the ethos of the profession. "Anybody who aims at a 40-hour week would be well-advised to follow some other vocation," suggested Dr H. Selwyn Kenrick in a letter to the New Zealand Herald that implied junior doctors had never had it so good.

For 15 years superintendent-in-chief of the Auckland Hospital Board and a former army doctor who had become a respected general practitioner, Dr Kenrick harked back to an earlier and even more authoritarian era. Describing his training at Dunedin Hospital in the South Island in the 1920s, he recalled that he had been one of just eight house surgeons (all junior doctors) in a 250-bed hospital. All of them had to live in the hospital – there were no provisions for married house surgeons. If he wanted to go into town for any reason, even a haircut, he was required to arrange for another doctor to cover for him in the hour or so he was absent from the ward.

His salary was £100 a year.

In short, he concluded, his own experience "indicates how greatly conditions have improved during the past 50 years."

Much of this kind of criticism missed the point though. Howie's ginger group had made it crystal-clear the campaign was not about a 40-hour week or anything remotely like it. Rather, it was simply a way of fixing a ceiling from which overtime could be calculated. He wanted to put a value on the number of extra hours worked. If hospital boards had to pay a fair price for hours above 40, they would eventually come to realise it made financial sense to hire more staff rather than continue working their junior doctors to the bone.

It took the best part of a year of battles with politicians and civil servants, hospital administrators and senior medical staff (of which a minority were supportive), but eventually the Howie campaign achieved a partial victory. This took the form of an interim deal that guaranteed compensatory payments after 40 hours, plus some extra leave including for cases of bereavement. These were of course exactly what the rest of the nation's workforce expected as of right.

At first the deal was based only on a temporary agreement, pending a full report into junior doctors' conditions. Previous campaigns had failed at this final hurdle, but on this occasion the report confirmed what the junior doctors had been saying all along, namely their working conditions were insupportable. And it led to arrangements that established an important principle of payment for overtime. For every hour worked above 40 to a maximum of 60, junior doctors would be paid five percent of the rate they had earned in the first 40. And for every hour between 60 and 84, they would be rewarded with ten percent of the amount paid in the first 40.

It wasn't a lot of money. In fact the payments would soon be jokingly described as "undertime". Yet a long-held and indefensible practice – that of extra work being provided for nothing -- had been overturned. "The recognition of overtime was the great victory," remembers Howie today.

Still, the battle to win a maximum 80-hour week, crucial in the campaign, had been comprehensively lost. Junior doctors were still required to work longer than 80 hours a week, and sometimes way longer. Not only were they still being overworked, they were expected to treat seriously ill patients in a sleep-deprived state.

This was the issue that had lain dormant for the previous decade – and for decades before that -- and it was the one that the junior doctors in the biggest city in New Zealand now intended to redress.

Cooper and his rebels had talked at length with Howie and others who had stuck their heads above the parapet, and learned a great deal about the deviousness of hospital administrators, politicians, civil servants and even members of their own profession. They would put these insights to good effect as they embarked on their own campaign.

Chapter three

A danger to the patients

All too soon it transpired that the junior doctors had picked the worst possible time for people on the government payroll to demand what amounted to a pay rise. While the new government was certainly committed to address workers' rights, as Cooper and his colleagues had assumed, it was not particularly the rights of working doctors that it had in mind. Additionally, the government's freedom to address any issues at all, whatever their merit, was greatly limited by how they might affect the public purse.

In early 1985, New Zealand's small and vulnerable economy was moribund. Global watchdogs such as the International Monetary Fund and Organisation for Economic Cooperation and Development were proposing that the new government undertake an urgent programme of fiscal reform, which most certainly did not include a round of inflationary, catch-up wage hikes. As the price of their continuing support, New Zealand's international lenders were insisting on disciplined management of the public finances.

The nation had endured three and a half years under the yoke of the infamous "freeze" imposed by ousted prime minister, the autocratic Sir Robert "Piggy" Muldoon. A chartered accountant by training, he had devised the heavy-handed regime as a response to a nearly calamitous bout of runaway inflation and clamped an iron hand on increases in prices, wages, interest rates and dividends. Like similar policies applied elsewhere, it had failed to address the nation's underlying economic problems and the economy had shrunk steadily for years. In Muldoon's final year in power, unemployment exceeded five percent in a country that historically prided itself on providing a job for nearly everybody who wanted one. Most importantly though, the economy was overborrowed and underperformed.

With few precedents to guide the government in the reform of a fragile and heavily regulated economy, it was unsure how to proceed. After all, Labour had been out of power for nearly a decade. The new hands on the helm did recognise though that central bargaining

-- the long-standing, rigidly controlled, state-run system of fixing wages and conditions for a highly unionised workforce -- had irretrievably broken down.

But what to put in its place? Not only was the government feeling its way, the nation's senior civil servants had dutifully attempted to run a red tape-bound economy for the best part of a decade and were out of their depth in what promised to be a market-based replacement.

To advance their cause in this highly fluid situation, Cooper and his committee knew the junior doctors had to pull together. But they also knew that one of the main reasons for earlier failures to improve junior doctors' circumstances was the inherent weakness in their own organisation. Although their representative national body, the New Zealand Resident Medical Officers Association, occasionally met to discuss pressing issues, it had always been difficult for succeeding committees to take a long-term view on them -- and certainly not on such fundamental matters as working hours and overtime that required concerted and sustained nationwide action.

The main reason for this structural weakness was the very nature of junior doctors' work – they were often on the move. As their careers progressed, they shifted to different hospitals within New Zealand or overseas, which made it difficult or impossible to make a commitment to a campaign. It had long been standard practice for the leadership of the regional and national organisations to change on an annual basis, which clearly did nothing for continuity.

The only way to mount an effective campaign, the Auckland rebels concluded, was to effectively take over the national body and run everything from Auckland, albeit with central support. After all, most of the previous campaigns to seek redress had originated from Auckland.

There were other reasons for the dismaying run of failures. Most junior doctors were already overworked and disinclined to throw themselves into a battle that required months of after-hours toil, and especially one whose outcome was highly uncertain. They also lacked a seat at the negotiating table. All matters affecting them, including pay and conditions of work, were dealt with on their behalf by the New Zealand Medical Association (NZMA), the doctors' principal organisation. More detrimentally, issues relevant to junior doctors were not considered separately but as part of a job lot with those of the specialists.

In these circumstances it was pretty much inevitable that the considerations of junior doctors came a poor second to those of their superiors.

And then there was the Department of Health. Previous campaigners had come up against formidable opposition from this ministry, which had always been able to muster a seasoned team of negotiators who could toss the ball around as long as they liked. Unlike the junior doctors, they weren't going anywhere and they had developed a time-honoured tactic based on wearing out the opposition, albeit with disarming courtesy.

Given the size of the odds against them, it was hardly surprising that no less than sixteen attempts to reform working conditions in the previous twenty years had been short-lived, including two in the late sixties and four in the seventies. The only exception was the partially successful Gordon Howie-led campaign a whole decade earlier. In total, fifteen campaigns had fallen flat on their face despite the best of intentions.

Despite these seemingly insurmountable odds, the rebels had every confidence they would win. "We were firebrands and we had huge energy," remembers Cooper.

All the rebels were committed. One of the main lieutenants in the Auckland committee was vice-president Boyd Swinburn, who was in the unusual position for a penurious, overworked registrar of being married with three children. Training in gastro-enterology, a specialty concerned with the digestive system, Swinburn was driven by "a hatred of injustice," as he vehemently puts it even after this length of time. Fortunately, he had passed most of his specialist exams the year before and was in a position to help organise the campaign – "it would have been impossible otherwise," he recalls. Unusually, his own senior doctors were generally supportive of him taking up the cudgels on behalf of their juniors.

Helping run the back room was John Mawson who somehow managed to combine his medical duties with volunteer service in New Zealand Army's elite SAS division, roughly the equivalent of the Green Berets, as well as running marathons in whatever was left of his spare time. Despite the pressure of studies, it was not uncommon for students at medical school to join the Medical Corps of the army through a special university unit. Not only did they earn some much-needed extra pay, they got to eat in the officers' mess where the meals were far superior to the food dished up in university residences. Mawson took the army more seriously than most, attending six week-long courses and even throwing himself into the rigours of basic training during summer holidays.

"I don't quite remember when, but I got this idea of becoming the SAS's Medical Officer," Mawson remembers. "I could have landed the appointment straight from the university's medical unit after I graduated but I wanted to be on an equal footing with the men, so I decided to do the selection course while I was still studying. When I passed that, I did the SAS training during weekends and holidays." A dedicated volunteer, Mawson even took three months off from his studies to live in barracks.

As well as being one of the fittest doctors on the planet, Mawson was highly organised. Indeed he had to be if he were to squeeze all these activities into his studies. Thus he was an ideal candidate to take charge of much of the backroom duties. And like Swinburn, he was fired up by the blatant unfairness of the position in which junior doctors found themselves. "The social injustice of the situation – for the patients, me and my colleagues, made the decision to get involved a no-brainer," he says.

The grand plan was for Swinburn to share the negotiating duties with Cooper while Mawson shouldered most of the publicity including writing, printing, folding and posting of the RMOA's monthly newsletter. Working with Mawson behind the scenes was trainee neurologist Elizabeth Walker, the only woman in her department in this fast-developing specialty.

Having learned a lot from the Howie campaign, which had failed to drum up much support in the South Island, the committee recognised the backing of junior doctors in the southern part of the country would be crucial rather than just from those in the hardest-pressed hospitals in the North Island. And they particularly needed Dunedin on their side. Most Scottish of New Zealand's four main cities, it had long been one of the least militant, perhaps because it was located so far from Auckland. Fortunately, in 1985 the junior doctors' president there was the highly principled and determined Paddy Dewan. Of Irish heritage, he saw medicine as a mission that started and ended with the patient and he had little patience with anything, bureaucracy in particular, that got in the road. When these views once made the local press, he immediately incurred the disapproval of senior management, who seemingly preferred to shoot the messenger rather than face the need for reform.

"It was inferred that I was a trouble-maker," he recalls. "It seemed they wanted an argument rather than go through a collaborative process with all stakeholders." As soon as he learned what the campaign was about, Dewan assured Auckland of his association's unwavering support.

Right from the start the Auckland committee regarded the civil servants from the Department of Health as the main opposition. "The junior doctors' leaders including Gordon Howie from ten and twenty years before told me not to trust the negotiators from the ministry," remembers Cooper. "They said they would try to delay us at every stage so they could deplete our energy. These officials knew our lives rotated around clinical obligations and they relied on the fact that eventually we'd just fade away."

As the committee laid the groundwork, Howie's experience proved particularly helpful. After all, his campaign had achieved more success than any other. The clear message that Howie gave to the new boys was that they must keep their feet on the necks of the ministry officials or they would lose momentum. In the mid-1970s Howie and his colleagues had run into one delaying tactic after another as they found himself on the side lines of a four-way slanging match between hospital boards, government and the opposition, and NZMA, none of the four being prepared to accept responsibility. The hospital boards blamed the government for cutting funds while the government blamed the hospitals for starving medical services in favour of administrative resources. "Whenever there is a cut-back in funds, it is the doctors and nurses who are reduced. I wonder why this is the case?" the health minister at that time, Tom McGuigan, grumbled to the media, implicitly revealing the yawning gulf in relations between government and the hospital system.

As Howie reminded the new rebels, for months on end he had great difficulty in even getting people in authority to talk to him. Hospital administrators, who had the ear of the senior doctors, appeared to regard the junior doctors as a nuisance. And the health minister had refused to agree to an appointment for almost a year. Eventually, a frustrated Howie had decided to take direct action – in short, a strike. Nor did he mince his words: "The minister won't do anything, the hospital board won't do anything."

In his briefings to his successors, Howie also stressed the importance of getting the media onside. During his campaign the nation's newspapers regularly ran articles about punishing hours for junior doctors, long queues of patients in A&E, and the general wear and tear on doctors' families. One Sunday tabloid sympathetically quoted an unnamed junior doctor -- "I just eat, sleep and work."

Cartoonists had a field day. One sketched a nurse holding up a single bottle of blood as she issued a warning to a horrified patient: "You'd better make this lot last, Mr. Wilby." Another depicted a bed-ridden man protesting at a woman visitor who had brought her son, a boy scout, into the ward. "I don't care how many first aid badges her boy's got, he's not volunteering to help out on me," he yelled.

Despite his conviction that the system had to change, Cooper was an accidental president of the Auckland association. "I got volunteered", he remembers somewhat ruefully. "But I knew that something just had to be done." Astonishingly in view of the conditions that the Howie campaign had exposed a decade earlier, he had found that the physical and emotional demands on junior doctors had increased during the intervening years rather than, as might be expected, the other way around.

Cooper had just taken up a post in Auckland Hospital with the long-term ambition of specialising in anaesthesiology after slogging away down the ranks as a house surgeon, working his way through many different specialised rotations that involved inordinately long hours. Although, as the son of a general practitioner, he had been forewarned about the rigours of a house surgeon's job and thought he was prepared for the worst. Instead he'd been shocked by the work load piled on him and his colleagues. He'd also been disappointed by the sometimes half-hearted supervision offered by seniors. More helpful had been the slightly more experienced junior doctors such as the registrars -- but they were run off their feet too and couldn't spare much time on supervision and advice.

Although Cooper was enjoying his new post – occasionally the seniors in anaesthesia might give the juniors a day off after a particularly arduous night, he still believed the time had come to redress matters, if only for the benefit of future junior doctors.

The memories of the boot camp years would never leave him though. "The work was non-stop, especially in the evenings," he recalls. At Green Lane Hospital on the other side of the city, for instance, a junior doctor covering general surgery in the early 1980s was required to work in one of three teams that had responsibility for a specific ward as well as to provide relief in other wards when the demand was high enough. There were four in each team – two consultants (senior doctors or specialists), a surgical registrar (a junior doctor starting to specialise), and a house surgeon (a junior doctor in his first two years).

The standard hours for junior doctors were 7.30am until 5.30pm five days a week, giving a basic 50-hour week. While there was generally time enough to snatch a meal and a couple of coffee breaks during these shifts, there was little or no chance of escaping for a nap. On the rare occasions they could grab an hour or two's sleep, they would generally retire to a small room, containing only a bed that was shoe-horned into a corner of the ward, close to the patients. Some hospitals offered a residence, like a cheap motel, that might be hundreds of metres away from the wards but where the junior doctors could at least get a meal and have a chat with colleagues.

But these were just the daylight shifts. Even that was a misnomer because, starting at 5.30pm and ending at 7.30am when the next team came on, the "daylight shift" ran right through the night. During evenings and weekends each team also took turns in covering all the acute wards. As for the weekend shifts, they were pretty much endless. They began at 7.30am on the Saturday and went through until 7.30am on the following Monday, giving a total of 48 hours. When the weekend shifts were added to the 50 week-day hours, it meant most junior doctors still ground their way through more than 90 hours of toil in a week.

In short, little had changed since the time of the Howie campaign.

It might be argued that these were only *rostered* hours and not necessarily all *working* hours. Certainly, there could be some respite from the pressure but this depended on the hospital. While some wards experienced quiet periods, most of them were busy nearly all the time and junior doctors generally spent the greater part of their shifts playing catch-up with cases. In smaller, often less well-equipped regional hospitals the workload could be just as heavy – and sometimes heavier -- because doctors had to cover more wards and deal with a greater variety of illness and trauma.

Perversely, the most-feared time of all was Monday morning when, in theory, the punishing weekend shift was meant to come to an end. Senior doctors had however a habit of button-holing their junior colleagues before they could slip out of the hospital with the dreaded words: "I've got a very interesting case you should look at."

Although the specialists could not insist they stay on after the Monday morning rounds were over, few juniors would dare reject such an invitation. If they valued their careers, they just bit the bullet and faced up to another ten hours on their feet. And it often did. When these voluntary Monday duties were added to the total of the entire weekend, a junior doctor could easily end up working 58 hours straight.

When everything was taken into account, it meant the rostered working week was merely a curtain-raiser for the main event. If the junior doctor was lucky enough not to be down for the 48-hour weekend shift (followed by the strong possibility of a ten-hour daylight one on Monday), a normal week meant 78 hours on the wards – that is, 50 daylight hours and 28 "evening" ones. Yet, astonishingly, doctors rostered for the weekend might end up doing 112 hours during the entire week – that is 50 daylight hours, 14 evening hours and 48 weekend hours – before turning around and starting the next week with another 10-hour daylight shift.

It could be argued that juniors had some time to recuperate from these punishing rosters during their statutory holidays, but there was a problem here too. They were often refused permission to take them on the grounds they could not be spared. This would become a bone of contention in the coming negotiations.

Inevitably, the limits of mind and body were reached. Even Mawson, who specialised in feats of endurance with the SAS, sometimes feared he was permanently wrecking his health. In one epic seven-day roster he clocked a superhuman 132 hours that was composed of four days and nights when he was on-call – that is, available over a 24-hour period, plus three 12-hour non-stop days during which he conducted a five-hour operation among other surgery.

Some disciplines were more exhausting than others. The greatest demands were usually made on the surgical, obstetrics and general medical wards – the orthopaedic house surgeon and registrar often got no sleep at all during an entire weekend. Other specialties might be less gruelling such as dermatology and psychiatry, which rarely produced acute cases that would keep junior doctors on their feet for 24 hours or more.

Punishing though it was on men, the system was even harder on women. Those who had an aptitude for one of the more challenging specialties such as surgery were often obliged to opt for a less onerous one, simply because it was impossible for them to do the required hours and still have a family.

In terms of remuneration, the more senior registrars (still junior doctors although some could have up to ten years experience) were particularly hard done by. Because they had to work exceptionally long hours, their salaries could easily approach those of the junior consultants – the tutor specialists -- who occupied several rungs higher up the professional ladder. This happened because, thanks to the Howie campaign, they were paid overtime – or rather, as we've seen, "undertime". Although the extra pay wasn't much, it was enough to threaten the incomes of junior consultants, which was considered unacceptable. So after a certain number of overtime hours was reached, a pay ceiling was imposed on the senior registrars. The result was that they ended up working for free once they reached this threshold.

Statistics did not tell the full story either. High as they were, the *number* of hours that junior doctors worked failed to convey the *intensity* of those hours. Because of the frequency of emergencies, the emotional pressure was particularly severe. The condition of an acutely ill patient might suddenly deteriorate. New cases would arrive with bowel blockages, ruptured appendices or other serious issues demanding immediate attention. Heart attacks and strokes were routine. Many patients were the victims of violence – deep stab wounds, severe concussion, broken limbs. Others were brought in with serious injuries sustained in sport. Drug addicts often arrived with their vital organs shutting down from overdoses.

In New Zealand acute medicine had its own idiosyncrasies. On the bright side there were hardly any gunshot victims, unlike in the United States as some junior doctors would discover when they went there for further training. But there were many severe injuries resulting from car crashes and alcohol-fuelled violence. In fact the two often went together.

Routinely faced with such traumatic cases, junior doctors had to quickly develop nerves of steel. In his first week covering a 500-bed regional general hospital, Peter Saunders remembers having to deal with seriously injured victims of a major road accident not long after he had graduated. As he would recall years later in a blog in Britain's Christian Medical Fellowship journal, he and another junior were the only doctors on duty when their patients turned up in ambulances, all of them in need of urgent attention. Of the four males involved, one suffered a cardiac arrest in the resuscitation room soon after he arrived.

"We were able to intubate, rehydrate and cardiovert him before the more senior staff arrived," Saunders recalled. Unfortunately, the patient would later die from serious multiple injuries.

The second victim needed an emergency tracheotomy for an obstructed airway, this operation being performed by more senior doctors who hurried into the hospital in the nick of time. The third male was flown out to a larger and better equipped hospital for emergency neurosurgery. And the fourth suffered a head injury from which he later recovered.

As one case after another was piled on overworked junior doctors, it was inevitable that mistakes were made. It wasn't the more routine procedures where things went wrong, such as hammering in a steel rod in surgery to stabilise a fractured bone, diagnosing a fracture on an X-ray, or stitching up a wound. Mistakes were more likely to be made in cases that required judgement, finesse and concentration at a time when physical and mental powers had fallen far below their peak.

As exhaustion deepened, the mind could play tricks. Some remember jumping out of bed and hurrying to a ward in the middle of the night only to be told they had never been called. They had imagined it. Others say they were virtually sleep-walking around the hospital, using all their energy just to stay on their feet. Neurologist Elizabeth Walker, who would take over some of the secretarial tasks in the backroom of the rebellion, recalls a shift that began on a Friday morning and did not finish until Monday night, an incredible 72-hour tour of duty in which she snatched just four hours sleep.

"At the end I was incapable of anything, even writing up my notes about a patient," she says.

Sometimes the consequences of marathon shifts bordered on the ridiculous. In the early hours of one morning, Mawson was admitting an elderly woman in the emergency area of the surgical ward. As he sat on the edge of her stretcher, jotting down notes about her medical history, he fell asleep. Jolting awake, he started again but with the same result. After he had dozed off for the third time, the woman suggested: "Why don't you get a few hours sleep, doctor? Then come back and finish. I'll be okay where I am."

He took her advice and went off for a nap, but this and similar incidents served as a warning. "The long gruelling hours affected my performance to the point where I didn't think I was safe to work with patients," he recalls.

And that, finally, was what motivated Cooper and his colleagues. At a certain level of exhaustion the ringleaders of the campaign had no doubt they had become dangerous.

Chapter four

The gauntlet is thrown

In early May, within five months of Cooper and his committee taking over the reins of the Auckland branch of the Resident Medical Officers Association (RMOA), a strong turnout of 200 members voted for a stop-work meeting. They wanted it to take place as soon as possible.

This was a big step into the unknown but, as Cooper had explained, direct action was the only way they could drag the hospital administration to the negotiating table. He had tried to raise with the management their issues of pay and working conditions — specifically, decent overtime rates and a limit to total hours worked — but repeatedly ran into a stone wall. "We won't get anywhere going through the normal channels," he told members.

The committee was pleasantly surprised by the level of militancy shown by the attendance at what was, after all, only a preliminary meeting. "I don't think any of us expected the degree of support for change that we found," Mawson would write later in his meticulously maintained diary.

As soon as the meeting broke up and the junior doctors returned to the wards, Cooper and his inner circle drafted a formal statement of the intention to stop work and arranged to have it circulated among members for approval. He also wrote to the presidents of the regional associations explaining what the Auckland branch was doing and asking for their help by canvassing for support among their own members.

As soon as the formalities were completed, Swinburn and Mawson sought an appointment with the medical superintendent at Auckland Hospital, a certain Dr. Leslie Honeyman, a Scot who had emigrated to New Zealand seven years earlier. Dr. Honeyman had done the hard yards in his youth and had little sympathy with what he appeared to see as a rebellion. Admitted to his office, the pair handed him the stop-work notice, as they were required to do. They remember the date -- May 23, a Thursday. "It was worth the trip to see Dr. Honeyman go pale," Mawson later recorded.

The stop-work notification was a turning point, as the committee well knew. They had thrown down the gauntlet and there was no going back. The furthest the Howie campaign had gone was to refuse to treat non-urgent cases such as infected tonsils and varicose veins, or to work no longer than 40 hours. Having got the better of that rebellion, in the intervening years the hospital management and board had clearly assumed that the junior doctors could be fobbed off ad infinitum.

But now the wheel had turned and the board was unsure how to react.

A sympathetic media jumped on the story. Top-rating current affairs programme Close Up followed Swinburn around the wards during an entire 36-hour shift that started in the morning and finished at the end of the next day, with almost no respite. For viewers the programme must have been a revelation. As the shift wore on, an increasingly exhausted-looking Swinburn was shown hurrying from case to case, several of them matters of life-and-death. Whenever the reporter was able to snatch a few minutes to sit him down for interviews, Swinburn's beeper would go off and he would hurry off to another case.

The documentary left an overwhelming impression of a team of young male and female doctors being inundated with cases – 45 in fact during the shift, most of which Swinburn had to see twice. As the most senior of the junior doctors, Swinburn was required to assume the biggest burden. "Are you tired? "the reporter unnecessarily asked towards the end of the shift. "Of course I'm tired", a haggard-looking Swinburn responded.

The Close Up team also interviewed an unsympathetic Dr. Honeyman who gave the impression of being largely unaware of how hard his junior staff was being pushed. When the reporter corrected him about the length of their shifts, the medical superintendent promptly switched tacks and made an observation about how valuable was the training they got during these long hours. In this, his views reflected those of most of the senior medical staff who appeared to believe junior doctors were fortunate to be getting so much experience.

The documentary became compulsory viewing for junior doctors – and probably many of the senior doctors too – and served to make the Auckland group even more militant. Around the same time, current-affairs radio conducted an interview with Cooper along similar lines while newspapers ran headlines about how junior doctors were being unfairly exploited and generally worked to exhaustion.

Thereafter events moved quickly, the committee being determined to maintain momentum. Precisely 359 junior doctors turned out right on schedule for the stop-work meeting on a wet day -- "not bad out of a total 420 in the Auckland region," noted Mawson in his diaries. The attendance voted overwhelmingly in support of all the resolutions that summarised the Auckland committee's campaign.

It was on the issue of extreme fatigue and its consequences that the rebels chose to draw a line in the sand. In this, the limit on total working hours was the key. Although junior doctors recognised they had chosen a profession in which it was not feasible to expect a 40-hour week or even a 60-hour one, their case would be grounded on the fundamental silliness and irresponsibility of imposing on them 90 hour-plus working weeks. As they argued, not only were punishing hours inherently counterproductive, they threatened the welfare of patients and left the doctors dangerously exposed to legal redress if things went wrong.

Right on cue, a case had occurred two months earlier in the resuscitation ward at North Shore Hospital when an exhausted junior doctor gave 400 milligrams of Lignocaine, eight times the recommended dose, to a patient who had suffered a cardiac arrest. The patient died and the police became involved. Were it not for the committee hastily organising medical representation at considerable expense, the incident could have spelled the end of the doctor's career. Most of the junior doctors in Auckland had heard of the case and it made them even more convinced they were on the right track.

By now, the Aucklanders had also persuaded the rest of the regional committees to throw their weight into the campaign. With Paddy Dewan's Dunedin group in the forefront, the other associations overwhelmingly backed the Aucklanders during a six-hour meeting in Wellington in late May. Debated in a series of brainstorming sessions in hospital canteens, coffee bars, restaurants and individuals' apartments during breaks from the wards, the battle lines had been built around three fundamental changes for junior doctor's working conditions: the right to independent negotiations in the future, reduced working hours – a maximum of 16-hour days and 72-hour weeks, and genuinely higher overtime pay rather than the much-resented "undertime".

The rebels knew the issue of the 16-hour day would be highly contentious and resisted by the hospitals. But they considered this to be only common sense when seen from the perspective of the welfare of both patient and doctor. It was also a blocking move, expressly designed to prevent junior doctors, who might have already worked 24 hours straight, from feeling obliged to stay on for the next day as well if they were "invited" to do so by the specialist.

The 72-hour week was a back-stop. If they could make that stick, hospital management could not then insist that junior doctors line up for one 16-hour day after another until they eventually ended up working 90 hours or longer, as was happening at that time. If they didn't win that one, nothing would have been gained and the entire campaign would go down as another failure.

Fundamentally, it all came down to maximum hours – that is, for each shift and each week.

The committee was also keenly aware that flexibility must be built into the arrangements. After all, acute illness does not respect the clock. And so it had been agreed that the 72-hour week should be seen as the *average* maximum over the full month rather than a fixed maximum to be observed in every week. If junior doctors were required to work, say, 76 hours in a particularly demanding week, they would be happy to do so on condition their hours were reduced proportionately during the rest of the month.

These numbers logically led to the next issue -- formal arrangements for genuine overtime. Their own experiences and those of earlier campaigners had convinced the rebels that hospital boards had to be forced to hire more junior doctors. And if overtime was paid at a rate that made virtually unlimited hours of work by a small team of junior doctors uneconomic, the boards would finally recognise it made sense to hire more doctors to plug the manpower gap. There had to be a tipping point, in short, at which the employment of more staff would save the hospitals money.

Thus overtime rates became the key to the solution. To put it plainly, the doctors had to jack up the rates to a high enough level to discourage the hospitals from paying them. At least the campaign started with one advantage -- it did not have to negotiate the *principle* of payment for overtime rates, which had been secured by the Howie campaign a decade earlier.

Before they went into battle with the Department of Health, the Aucklanders made a crucial decision. They would hire a professional negotiator. Having learned once again from the Howie campaign when the junior doctors had attempted to do all the bargaining on their own and come off second-best, Cooper had gone looking for an individual who was familiar with how the system worked in the capital city and who had a successful track record. In short, a seasoned advocate.

By this stage the Auckland committee had managed to raise the funds to bankroll the campaign. The nationwide membership had responded to a request for a voluntary $100 donation per person and handed over a collective $100,000 within a few days. It was an unprecedentedly large sum that attested the degree of dissatisfaction among the country's junior doctors – and it was enough to hire the professional negotiator.

"Which union's got the best deal lately?" Cooper asked his colleagues. The answer was pretty much immediate: "The airline pilots."

Cooper found his man in Rod Trott, a specialist in industrial law who had handled a string of high-profile negotiations over pay and conditions including, most recently, the pilots. Members of a powerful union, the pilots were employed mainly by government-owned Air New Zealand, the national carrier, and they had just agreed a handsome salary package. Most importantly, Trott was closely acquainted with New Zealand's home-grown and eccentric system of arbitration. Having studied at the London School of Economics and later worked in the Federation of Labour, the unions' umbrella organisation, alongside its veteran president Sir Tom Skinner before branching out into professional negotiation under his own shingle, he had represented a variety of clients including waterfront workers and traffic controllers as well as the pilots – and won substantial awards on their behalf. Although Trott had never taken on a brief from the medical profession, he knew who mattered and who didn't in the capital city.

He was an insider in a town that thrived on relationships in the corridors of power.

The health minister at the time was Dr Michael Bassett, not a medical doctor but an historian who had earned his degree in American history while studying at USA's Duke University. He had been handed the hot seat by prime minister David Lange, a warm-hearted socialist who represented one of the nation's poorer constituencies and had made election speeches about the need for reform of the health system.

Proud of the fact that New Zealand, a pioneering nation in social welfare, had established a Department of Health nineteen years before Britain, Bassett took over the portfolio with the highest of intentions. Sitting on the opposition benches for nine long years, he had been frustrated at the way the system had been run down under the former government. For him, as it was for his party, the provision of an excellent health service was a founding principle of government.

Bassett's was a notoriously politically sensitive portfolio. Previous ministers had been caught in the crosshairs of a public that wanted cradle-to-the-grave healthcare at no cost to itself (patients did not pay for medical services in state-run hospitals), and of highly trained doctors who expected remuneration commensurate with their skills as well as world-class technology with which to practise them. The New Zealand Medical Association had rarely enjoyed a cordial relationship with governments of any stripe.

Health was also a complex ministry, with many arms and legs. No less than 104 different bodies reported to the minister, some of which had been in existence for decades and assumed unfettered right of access to Bassett as well as to the health budget. And here was the problem – Bassett had a paltry amount in his war chest. Because of the parlous state of the economy, the government came to office strapped for cash and ill-equipped to repair what the new minister described as "a decade of neglect" in the hospitals.

On the bright side the new minister seemed disposed to do what he could. In a speech entitled Cracks in the Health Services, Bassett identified a general shortage of nurses, specialists and, encouragingly, junior doctors. "Some hospitals seem to be operating with a lower junior doctor establishment than the workload would justify," he said in an implicit acknowledgement of the problem he would soon face.

Once he became acquainted with his brief, Rod Trott felt he was on familiar ground. During his campaign on behalf of the airline pilots he had seen how hierarchical and authoritarian systems had built up within the aviation industry and how hard they were to break down. "It was a colonial model of rewards that was based on not questioning your superiors even when you knew they were acting unsafely," he would explain, neatly encapsulating some of the resentments that lay behind his new clients' case.

The hospital system was certainly hierarchical and authoritarian. The administrators had proved time and again they were almost systemically unsympathetic to the junior doctors' cause. And with limited budgets to deploy, they were firmly opposed to any reforms that increased the running costs of the hospitals. As far as they were concerned, severe financial constraints justified their determination to manage hospitals as cheaply as they could, even if that included running junior doctors into the ground.

There was another incentive to leave things as they were -- the hospitals had long enjoyed the benefit of a rate of productivity that was off the scale. As we have seen, the system was based on virtually unlimited hours of overtime that were rewarded on a diminishing scale – the longer junior doctors worked, the less they earned. Here surely was a convenient and cheap method of employing manpower that piled a lot of work onto the shoulders of a few. So clearly, there were powerful financial reasons for administrators to retain a system that delivered so much for so little.

The general attitude of senior doctors to the campaign varied. Some were quietly encouraging, others disapproving, and a few genuinely aghast. Some committee members were given veiled warnings that they were risking their careers. It was hard to ignore the fact that the consultants drew up the reports on junior doctors that went to the respective colleges where they hoped to specialise. An adverse remark or two could easily jeopardise their prospects in a highly competitive field. Nor was there any comeback against a hostile report such as the opportunity of seeking redress.

Some of the hostility stemmed from what was perceived as junior doctors' effrontery in attempting to reform a system that had been in place a long time – and one which the senior doctors had survived.

As things came to a head, the question of the "handover" began to crop up frequently. As we've seen, according to the prevailing view, especially in surgery, junior doctors should be available for as long as possible after a major operation in case the patient's condition deteriorated suddenly. Only when the patient was in a stable state should the handover to a new doctor occur. (By contrast physicians, who are specialists in cardiology and other non-operating disciplines, tended to be more relaxed about the issue.)

Overall, the campaign confronted a largely authoritarian system in which junior doctors' role was to listen and learn – and certainly not to question things. In her specialty of neurology, Walker had been on the receiving end of her fair share of snubs. When she once dared to venture a view on a patient, she was bluntly informed: "I'm not interested in your opinion."

As Trott planned his strategy, he took into account the way the long-standing, New Zealand-wide industrial relations system was disintegrating into what threatened to become a free-for-all. Founded on a Utopian sense of egalitarianism in which all the bureaucratic processes were rigidly defined, all the participants -- unions, employers organisations and government -- had long taken part in an annual joint exercise that resulted in the imposition of blanket, nationwide labour contracts on industries, individual employers and employees, regardless of whether these contracts were suitable or even affordable.

The system of industrial law was symptomatic of the way New Zealand governments had worked since the 1950s. New Zealanders had grown up under all-pervasive regulation that ranged from sky-high tariffs that blocked or greatly limited the entry of all kinds of goods and products such as automobiles, however useful and important they may be, or made them impossibly expensive for ordinary citizens to buy. Developed long before the arrival in power of the ousted Sir Robert Muldoon but perfected during his nine years in office, this highly restrictive and regulated economy had long been tolerated by New Zealanders.

Playwright and wit George Bernard Shaw had remarked on a visit to New Zealand in 1934 that New Zealanders lived in a communist society but didn't realise it. As late as the early seventies there was a standard jibe about pilots telling passengers "to put their watches back 20 years" before landing in New Zealand. And in the eighties, just as this system was crumbling, economists used to joke that New Zealanders should go to Albania to see what their country was once like.

Quite apart from opposition from within the hospital system to the junior doctors' demands, the new government was extremely wary. "There was a huge pent-up demand for wage increase," remembers health minister Bassett. "The junior doctors claim was just one of many in a massive pay round after more than three years of the wages and prices freeze."

Also, as far as the government was concerned, the junior doctors were a long way down the queue.

Chapter five

Impasse

As Cooper, Swinburn and Trott entered the offices of the Department of Health in downtown Wellington to face a formidable team of civil servants, their advocate whispered a warning: "This is going to be a marathon. Take a deep breath and settle down."

Privately, Trott was concerned that his clients were in so militant a mood that they might open negotiations by making demands that could not possibly be met. Their expectations for a quick and favourable result, he felt, were unrealistic and could torpedo the campaign almost before it had begun.

At Trott's suggestion the junior doctors had brought into negotiations another veteran unionist, Tony Neary. Greatly respected by some in the labour movement and reviled by others, he was an Irishman who hailed from County Mayo. He was also well-known to successive New Zealand governments that had come to respect – and fear -- his formidable bargaining skills. Neary had led the electrical workers union for most of his career while earning a reputation for taking highly principled stands, even if they upset leading lights in the union movement.

To his great credit, it was Neary who had fought the communist faction within the Federation of Labour in several bloody backroom battles. Twenty years earlier he had taken on the federation's leader, the former Marxist Fintan Patrick Walsh, known as the "Black Prince" for his glowering manner, in a libel case that had gone down in union folklore because it pitted the pro-Soviet far left against the pro-socialist right. New Zealand is a long way from the Kremlin but many a hard-line union boss had grown up on a diet of Marxist propaganda and become evangelists for the cause, even though the Soviet Union was turning into a ruthless and bloody dictatorship. Although Neary's side won this particular battle, it was a Pyrrhic victory because it earned him Walsh's undying enmity and rendered him persona non grata within the trade union establishment for years on end. (Much later, Neary would entitle his autobiography The Price of Principle.)

Now in his mid-sixties and approaching retirement, Neary was once again outside the union Pale. He had just quit the federation over its failure to negotiate a better deal for its members following the end of the wages and prices freeze. As a result, as journalist Mathew Dearnaley would later recall in an obituary in the New Zealand Herald, Neary had been "snubbed by the Labour government, of whose party he was a member but which would deal only with the federation."

But here Neary was, supporting the junior doctors in a change of scene. And whether he was inside or outside the union movement, Neary was a good man to have on your side. He had just won his electrical workers a 15.5 percent pay rise and he had a lifetime of experience in the bureaucratic hornet's nest of the capital city. Officially, his role in the negotiations was to serve as a kind of mentor to the junior doctors, all of whom were novice negotiators, and bolster the numbers of a small team.

His presence came as a surprise to the officials, as did that of Trott. "When Trott and Neary walked into a roomful of negotiators with us, it changed the whole dynamics," recalls Swinburn. The department's negotiators suddenly realised they were up against professionals.

But once the civil servants recovered from their surprise, the junior doctors got the impression their opponents believed they were not playing by the rules. "They thought doctors should behave themselves and not do this sort of thing," Trott would recall. "And they hoped we'd just go away, as had happened before."

Nor were the officials particularly pleased to see Jeremy Cooper walking into the room because it was his father, Dr Michael Cooper, who had just taken their minister all the way to the High Court over another contentious issue.

Despite the best of intentions, Bassett had got off to a bad start. Because the nation's hospitals consumed nearly seven percent of the government's gross national expenditure, the minister was under heavy pressure to keep a tight lid on costs while still maintaining the quality of health services. (He was also fending off a pay claim from nurses, with other claims in the pipeline.)

Aiming to help children in poorer areas, he had imposed a fixed charge of a dollar on pharmaceutical prescriptions in the expectation that the resulting extra revenues would subsidise visits to general practitioners in disadvantaged neighbourhoods. "The government had limited resources and I wanted to get more bang for the buck in the health system," Bassett would explain after his retirement. The vehicle for the intended reform was an existing arrangement known as the children's General Medical Services (GMS).

The health minister could have run the extra money through the NZMA, but he did not trust the doctors' organisation to ensure the funds went to patients rather than into general practitioners' pockets. So the government imposed a cap on their fees, subject to annual adjustments.

The tactic immediately put the medical fraternity offside. Unhappy at what they saw as government meddling in their right to set their own fees, a three-strong ginger group of general practitioners led by Jeremy Cooper's father took the issue to the High Court, arguing that the health minister had breached the terms of the GMS. To Bassett's dismay, the High Court came down heavily against him.

"I got a thorough bashing," he recalled, albeit without rancour. "The judge threw the book at me." (It might also be argued that his officials gave him the wrong advice.)

The ruling meant the government had no alternative but to abandon the cap on general practitioners' fees, leaving the minister red-faced. It was however a short-lived bashing because the government slipped some fine print into the next budget that made the cap legal. Yet the incident served as a reminder that the medical profession was a tough foe who was prepared to take an issue all the way.

Simultaneously, the health minister was fighting off controversies on all sides. He had hardly got behind his desk when he became embroiled in the long-running anti-smoking debate between a combative medical profession, among other equally aggressive factions, and a tobacco industry fighting a rear guard action. In yet another example of the sensitivities of his portfolio, he had disappointed the former by decreeing that cigarette packets bear the warning "Smoking Endangers Health" when the NZMA had campaigned for the tougher "Smoking Kills" that had already been adopted by Australia.

At that stage the junior doctors' campaign probably seemed the least of the health minister's worries.

As soon as the negotiators sat down, Trott handed over the formal claim that the team had spent months drawing up. The document was carefully framed to highlight the single main imperative on which the junior doctors were determined that negotiations should be conducted. "I fashioned it around the overtime issue," he remembers. "We demanded steep overtime rates that we knew would force hospitals to organise junior doctors differently."

Although the officials were somewhat put out by the presence of professional negotiators, they could at least draw some comfort in the knowledge that proceedings would be conducted according to what they regarded as proper procedure. "I got a sense of their relief that at least someone who was an adult was on the junior doctors' side," recalls Cooper. "[They felt] there could only be a conclusion to these talks if they were dealing with a person with whom they were familiar – and that person was Rod."

Back in Auckland where he was coordinating the publicity, Mawson was coming to the same opinion. "We understood the medical world. And we also understood the broader injustice of the hours we were working and their impact it was having on our performance and on the patients, on learning and on our personal lives," he remembers. "But Rod understood the world of politics, business and negotiating. He recognised that the issue of hours was fundamentally a business proposition for the hospital boards. It was all about how cheaply they could deliver this medical service. We were neophytes in this world. Without Rod, we knew we'd be at a serious disadvantage."

As Trott expected, negotiations immediately stalled. Hardly had the talking started when the officials bluntly informed the junior doctors there would be no compromise on what was known as "the ceiling," the rates earned by the tutor specialists who occupied the next rank up the hospital hierarchy. This meant that, if any junior doctor working under the overtime rates proposed in the negotiating document ever reached the same income as these junior specialists, all subsequent hours would have to be done for free.

It took simple arithmetic to conclude the entire campaign would immediately collapse if this condition was accepted. After all, the whole point was to force the hospitals to pay higher overtime rates and coerce them into hiring more staff. If the health ministry's arbitrary ceiling was to be enforced, the junior doctors would have to settle for paltry increases in overtime and all would be lost at the very outset.

Throughout the next few meetings, despite Trott's repeated objections, the officials refused to budge. "The initial reaction was denial and avoidance," he remembers.

The junior doctors were up against a stone wall.

After discussions with his clients, the advocate elected to try another approach. Instead of bashing heads in face-to-face negotiations, he would try and outflank the department. Thereupon he began to arrange meetings with influential senior officials in government departments other than health. At these he explained the guiding principle behind the junior doctors' campaign. Trott's purpose was get in ahead of the health department officials and forestall them from misrepresenting things. In all these briefings he stuck to the same argument: patients' lives were at risk because they were being treated by chronically sleep-deprived doctors.

Although negotiations were proceeding at a snail's pace in Wellington, back in Auckland there was a fever of activity as Mawson, Walker and other helpers took charge of a host of backroom functions. "We were very much the supporting cast, marshalling the troops," Mawson remembers. There was a lot to be done – newsletters written and posted, records and minutes maintained, scores of letters and notes drafted, hundreds of phone calls made, meetings organised.

The issue of the junior doctors soon came to a head for the health minister. Bassett returned from an overseas trip in May 1985 that included a tour of hospitals in the United States, Europe and Australia only to find himself in the middle of a crisis that was uncomfortably close to the issues raised by the junior doctors' campaign. The media was suggesting that the deaths of three patients in the acute wards at Auckland's Middlemore Hospital, one of the biggest in the country, were significantly attributable to inadequate staff numbers.

Under pressure from all sides as opposition politicians jumped on the band wagon, the minister was obliged to open an enquiry. But if Bassett hoped its findings would let his department off the hook, he was quickly disabused. Although the report did not directly attribute the death of two of the patients to staff shortages, it did so in the case of the third, a child suffering from severe burns. In that unfortunate event, the report concluded, inadequate medical attention was a significant factor in the patient's demise. The explanation was that the staff shortage had been created by the absence on leave of two specialists.

Batting the controversy away, the minister in effect blamed hospital management for giving the specialists permission to be simultaneously off the wards. Yet the report did highlight the fact that competent staff was thinly spread in the acute wards of one of the nation's busiest hospitals. If the absence of just two specialists left a hospital critically exposed, there were clearly not enough doctors to go around.

Rude homecoming though it was, the minister's overseas trip had taught him a lot about health budgets. As he subsequently informed medical organisations in a series of briefings, health systems were struggling everywhere he went. Much wealthier countries than New Zealand were battling to meet mounting costs, mainly because of the expense of rapidly advancing technologies in areas such as anaesthetics, radiology and surgery, in fact across the entire hospital spectrum.

Ominously for the junior doctors' campaign, Bassett also reminded the medical fraternity that hospitals everywhere were struggling to pay qualified staff what they were worth – or, rather, what they thought they were worth. While acknowledging that more and more patients were landing in New Zealand's acute wards, and thereby adding to the burden borne by junior doctors, he said in so many words that his hands were tied.

"Demands for higher wages [in overseas hospitals], while often warranted, are compounding problems," Bassett declared in a thinly veiled warning that the government would not look sympathetically on generous pay hikes for junior doctors, or indeed for anybody else employed by the hospitals.

However a shortage of funds in the health system was one thing, the provision of urgent medical attention by half-asleep junior doctors another. And it was an issue that was coming to fore in other countries. In February of that year, a report in the New England Journal of Medicine concluded that "time pressures and sleep deprivation constitute the major stresses in residency training, adversely affecting the ability of residents to learn, the quality of medical care they deliver, and their ability to respond appropriately to urgent problems."

The issue of sleep-deprived doctors was turning into a global matter. The research published in the New England Journal of Medicine helped provoke a debate about patients' rights that raised difficult questions about inexperienced doctors being expected to deal with complex and urgent cases.

And then the Libby Zion affair landed like a thunderclap in American medicine.

Just 18 years old, Libby Zion was an aspiring journalist who lived at home with her father Sidney Zion, a combative newspaper columnist and former trial lawyer, and mother Elsa, a city official. The daughter had a history of depression and cocaine use. On the evening of March 4, 1984, she had fallen ill with flu-like symptoms. Her condition rapidly worsened and she began to convulse. Taken to New York Hospital for treatment, she was given a painkiller and a sedative and, to prevent her from harming herself as she thrashed about, she was strapped to her bed. Libby Zion died early the following morning of cardiac arrest, eight hours after admission.

Her parents were shocked, grief-stricken – and baffled. How could their daughter die so rapidly of what had seemed a minor ailment? Concluding that she had been fatally mistreated by exhausted junior doctors working without proper supervision, Zion and his wife sued New York Hospital and four doctors on the grounds of gross negligence. The case hit the headlines, once again raising disturbing and deep-seated issues about the conditions under which residents (junior doctors in America) worked as well as about the responsibilities piled on young shoulders.

Meantime in New Zealand, as negotiations dragged on, the health department appointed a working party to investigate junior doctors' conditions. As it happened, the findings would coincide closely with the conclusions reached by the report in the New England Journal of Medicine, noting for good measure that there had been little improvement. Indeed the main conclusion was that the position "remains very similar to that described in the Henley Report conducted four years earlier."

As far as the junior doctors were concerned, the report was an exercise in futility. It proved what everybody knew already and, as such, provided just another example of the health department's stalling tactics. Still, it did at least serve to bring the issue up to date and confirm the junior doctors' arguments.

Five main areas of concern were identified in the report. First, junior doctors were working punishing hours "often without interruption for periods of rest". Second, they were being remunerated at a decreasing rate of return for those extra hours. Third, they had trouble getting statutory leave (another issue Trott had laid on the table). Fourth, their work experience was poorly managed. Fifth, they felt they were taken for granted and had no say in their own working conditions.

Although no mention was made of salaries and pay rates because the researchers were specifically precluded from dealing with them, the conclusions were damning.

By contrast, the working party had looked at the Australian system and been impressed. As Swinburn and other junior doctors had already experienced during stints in hospitals on the other side of the Tasman Sea, there were important differences in Australia.

Their hospitals generally employed more junior doctors than comparably sized New Zealand ones. Hardly any junior doctors (interns in Australia) were rostered on 24-hour shifts because most hospitals ran a system of night residents who covered the wards between 11pm and dawn. The hours were also much shorter – between 40-48 hours in a basic working week – and significant penalty rates applied for overtime. Instead of the descending scale applying in New Zealand, Australian overtime rates actually *rose* the longer the doctors worked.

And importantly, A&E departments were better managed, functioning more as acute units rather than as admissions for all kinds of conditions that did not necessarily require emergency treatment.

Although different states in Australia had their own variations, the conditions were broadly similar right across the nation. In New South Wales, for instance, junior doctors could work up to 48 hours in one weekend, but they were handsomely rewarded for doing so. "Some registrars work extraordinarily long hours and attract very high levels of remuneration," the report would note.

As one study after another was making clear, the health minister was right. Hospitals in the western world, as in New Zealand, were struggling to function under increasingly fraught circumstances. Such was the demand for beds that people were being treated and discharged more rapidly than before. Consultants were running around with clipboards and recording turnover rates and bed availability, as though they were clocking occupancy levels in the hotel industry. The entire hospital system was in a state of relentless transition. However, the studies also showed that while just about everybody who worked in the system was under mounting pressure, junior doctors bore much more than their fair share.

In mid-1985, the first detailed survey of work and sleep patterns of New Zealand's junior doctors told the story. Commissioned by the RMOA to put hard numbers behind their campaign, it involved more than 1,000 house surgeons, senior house officers and "category one" registrars throughout New Zealand – that is, all those whose job descriptions required them to stay in the hospital during their rostered hours.

The findings were startling. Two thirds worked 75 hours a week (regular and on-call) and got less than five hours sleep a night. Some were rostered for as much as 57 hours at a stretch. In that entire stint they would be lucky to snatch a few hours rest. The hardest-working respondent in the survey clocked a Herculean 134 hours, which left less than five hours a day for sleeping, eating and studying.

In short, junior doctors had almost no life outside the hospital.

As the first methodical analysis of junior doctors' work load, the survey confirmed all the anecdotal evidence and what the media had been reporting. It also provided backing for the principles that underpinned the case. As Swinburn explains: "It put statistics on all the stories that were appearing in the media and was pivotal for the campaign."

When the survey was released, Swinburn followed up with a letter to the New Zealand Medical Journal that left no doubt the situation had become untenable, if only from the viewpoint of the patient. "The ability of junior doctors to detect abnormalities on ECGs, laboratory forms and other tests markedly decreases with sleep deprivation," he wrote. "Patient care must inevitably deteriorate." This observation also, of course, reflected research then being published in overseas journals.

Swinburn also alluded to the health risks run by young doctors, warning of well-established side-effects such as "psychological difficulties" that included depression and irritability and even dependence on drugs and alcohol that could lead to suicide. In support of the survey, he cited American research published two years earlier in the International Journal of Medical Education that came to a startling and thought-provoking conclusion: "Physicians, in short, are destroying themselves at twice the rate of the population they want to keep healthy."

As Trott continued to quietly lobby senior officials and ministers on the sidelines of the negotiations, meetings with the health department's officials became tedious exercises in stonewalling as they refused to budge on the all-important issue of the tutor specialists' pay ceiling. But as they realised this latest campaign was not going to fade away without something to take back to the supporters, the officials began to throw them small carrots that, they hoped, would bring things to an acceptable conclusion. These carrots mainly took the form of promises to undertake further research into their issues even though there was already a plethora of existing studies, most of which said more or less the same thing.

Tony Neary, the veteran negotiator, was proving invaluable. Not in the least intimidated by high-ranking civil servants and ministers, he never raised his voice or banged the table, preferring to play his cards close to his chest. He was so experienced in the subtleties of New Zealand's civil service that Cooper and Swinburn got the impression he could read the direction in which things were heading, almost as though he had his own compass.

"If he said we were being mucked around, he would quietly advise us to let them have it," remembers Cooper. "At other times he told us we were being offered something that would work, even if it wasn't clear to us. He was extremely constructive."

Still, the junior doctors had no doubt that the officials' strategy remained unchanged – that is, to outlast them. After all, the tactic had worked often enough before. And to be fair, they were defending a budget. Nearly all government ministers were under strict instructions to run a tight ship until the New Zealand economy could struggle back to its feet.

Bassett was following the script, firing regular broadsides at the hospitals. "The government is determined to control its expenditure and obtain efficiencies in all government-funded organisations," he warned them. "We look to you and to your boards to work with us in this exercise."

None of this looked particularly auspicious for the junior doctors' cause. However, with the assistance of Mawson and the backroom staff who fed stories to reporters, a sympathetic media kept the campaign in the headlines and put the health minister on the hook. Eventually, he identified three solutions to the "junior doctor problem," as he put it. First, there had to be an increase in the medical school intake. Second, an "aid programme" would import doctors from other countries to take up the slack until more doctors graduated in New Zealand. And third, there should be "a rearrangement of the rosters and workloads, which eases the burden on junior staff."

The last was pie in the sky – it was beyond anybody's ability to devise a roster that could turn one junior doctor into two. That left the first two solutions, both of which had some merit. The only problem was it would take anything from two to five years to make them happen and the junior doctors were not prepared to wait that long.

Chapter six

About the money

On July 26, nearly six months after the launch of their campaign, the junior doctors had a meeting with the health minister in Wellington. The atmosphere was highly charged.

Having been hauled before the highest court in the land over his scheme to improve medical care for poorer communities, Bassett did not welcome more agitation by the medical profession. Also, he remained determined to protect his precious health budget. In this, he was heartened by a pay claim that he and prime minister David Lange had just settled with the nurses without inflicting serious damage to it.

The junior doctors were proving a tougher nut to crack though. As he would record later in Working with David, a book about his relationship with the prime minister: "Meanwhile junior doctors, led by the son of one of the three GPs who had taken me to court over the child GMS, made life difficult for departmental officers, hospital boards and me."

It was the highest-level meeting so far, with no less than three ministers in the room as well as their advisers. In addition to Bassett, there was the minister for state services Stan Rodger and associate finance minister Richard Prebble. Rodger had one of the sharpest minds in the government and knew everybody who mattered in the capital city. A former president of the powerful Public Service Association, the union of civil servants, Rodger had the immensely complex job of leading negotiations with unions and employers in the post-freeze pay round and he was fighting off the Federation of Labour. The unions were pressing for a one-off general wage order that, they hoped, would give them the best possible result.

"But I was most anxious not to have a general wage order. I wanted negotiations," remembers Rodger. "The break-out from the freeze was tough stuff."

Although sympathetic to the junior doctors' case, Rodger was worried that a generous settlement with them would roll right through the government payroll and damage an economy that hadn't even begun a recovery. There were about 300,000 people on the payroll and nearly all of them were clamouring for fatter pay packets. The unexpected appearance of

Tony Neary, a well-known supporter of high settlements, did not make the minister any happier.

As for associate finance minister Richard Prebble, he was famously blunt. Also minister responsible for state-owned enterprises, he was a self-appointed watchdog of wasteful public expenditure, of which there were quite enough examples to raise his ire. Later, he would describe them in a memoir of his political life entitled *I've Been Thinking*.

If nothing else, the presence of no less than three senior ministers told the junior doctors that the campaign was turning into a problem for the government, just as Bassett would later acknowledge in his memoirs. It was certainly turning into a problem for the hospital boards who were being admonished to manage their budgets responsibly on the one hand while on the other wondering what would happen to their acute wards if the junior doctors were to walk off the job. So far, there had been just the one stop-work meeting, but the prospect of a strike hung ominously in the air.

The junior doctors were on the brink of exhaustion, Cooper and Swinburn in particular. They had been flying down to Wellington just about every week for negotiations, fruitless though they largely were, as well as conducting strategy-planning sessions with the national executive and their own team up in Auckland. In their few spare days, they were touring the nation's hospitals, sometimes in company with Mawson, where they discussed the developing situation with junior doctors. Although it was an unsettling situation to consider, the prospect of a nationwide strike was on the agenda in these discussions.

They just hoped it would never come to that.

Adding to the rebels' fatigue, their clinical duties were starting to weigh heavily on them. They could only get time away from the wards to run the campaign and sit down opposite ministry officials if their colleagues agreed to provide cover, a favour they did willingly despite their own massive workloads. But because the meetings in the capital took place between Monday and Friday, it meant that Cooper and Swinburn could fulfil their medical obligations only by working practically continuously during weekends to pay their colleagues back. This endless cycle of work and negotiations had been going on for months. Even when they could snatch a spare hour or two from the hospital, it was usually spent on campaign business.

Also, exams were looming. If they didn't pass these, the rebels knew they would never be granted entry into their desired specialties. The fate of Howie was well known. He had been rejected for his orthopaedics specialty despite excellent credentials and departed overseas to develop his skills rather than wait around another year to reapply in the hope his superiors had forgiven him.

An undercurrent of resentment was also becoming apparent in the hospitals. Although by no means universal, it was expressed by some hospital executives and members of the medical establishment, just as it had a decade earlier during the Howie campaign. (To this day, Howie can name the doctors who voiced their disapproval as well as those who went out of their way to provide support.) Some critics believed the young dissidents were letting down the profession by having the effrontery to pursue the campaign in the first place while others made it clear they were threatening a time-honoured system of practising medicine.

Various arguments were being mustered against what amounted to reduced hours, the chief of these being the continuing issue of the "handover". As senior doctors told Swinburn: "Continuity of care is the underlying foundation of looking after patients. The doctor who operates on a patient at 10 o'clock at night must be there at 3 o'clock in the morning when the complications occur. He knows the problems best."

The junior doctor did not buy this argument. As Swinburn pointed out to his superiors, the handover must inevitably happen at some point in the patient's recovery, simply because no doctor could stay on his feet for ever. "There comes a time when a doctor must go home and hand over the care of his patients to other covering doctors," he argued. "It's only a question of *when* to break the continuity, not *if* to break it." After all, he added, nurses worked fixed shifts and, although they were also crucial to a patient's well-being, they still had to release patients to the welfare of their replacements on the ward. This was, Swinburn said, a system that had stood the test of time.

But he also had a solution. Namely, he argued for a sufficient overlap of perhaps two hours between junior doctors leaving and their replacements arriving so that the latter could be fully briefed.

Another argument mounted by the hierarchy was the one pertaining to rosters. According to this, it would be impossible to devise rosters that could accommodate reduced hours, overlaps and everything else the junior doctors were proposing. "It's never been done," they argued in so many words.

But here again Swinburn had a response: "The benefits to the patients of shorter hours far outweigh any consequential logistic difficulties."

And finally, there was the economic argument. When administrators protested at the high cost of hiring more junior doctors, Swinburn mounted a thought-provoking moral argument: "The price of cotton went up when slavery was abolished. Did that deter Abraham Lincoln from his humanitarian principles?"

And that was a hard one to rebut.

The meeting with the ministers had hardly started when tempers began to fray. After months of deadlocked weekday negotiations followed by long weekend shifts on the wards, Cooper and Swinburn were in no mood to be fobbed off any longer with empty promises. But the minister was also losing patience.

"It's just about the money," Bassett accused them.

"You're totally wrong," Cooper shouted back.

Just before the situation deteriorated into a slanging match, Prebble banged the table with his fist. "Stop the nonsense," he ordered. "I haven't got time for this. I've got a country to run."

This was something of an exaggeration because Prebble was only associate finance minister, the actual finance minister being Roger Douglas whose attempts to fix the ailing economy had been dubbed "Rogernomics". He also held tightly to the nation's purse strings.

Prebble's intervention had the desired effect however. The protagonists sat back in their chairs, took a deep breath and the meeting got down to business. The sticking point was the same as it had been for months. With the backing of his officials, the health minister insisted that the government could not afford to agree to all the doctors' demands because of the financial burden it would impose on the hospitals and the damage it would do to his slim health budget.

In this, Bassett was looking over his shoulder. Finance minister Douglas had already made it clear to Bassett that he was extremely unhappy with the nurses' wage increase, modest though it was.

As Bassett would later write: "Despite our interventions, which undoubtedly reduced the amount they might have obtained, the cost of the nurses' settlement still horrified Douglas."

The ministers did make two concessions however. First, they agreed that no shift should exceed 16 hours straight, or 72 hours per week. And second, they offered two avenues for further negotiation of wages. As far as the ministers were concerned, this was a handsome offer.

The junior doctors saw it differently. First, the concessions were offered only "in principle". Second, there was no timetable for their implementation. And third, they failed to address the point.

Despite the health minister's comment, the campaign had never been about the wages. Also, the junior doctors knew the proposed limits on hours could not be enforced without the significant increase in overtime rates that would give the hospitals no option but to increase staff numbers as a cheaper option to paying the overtime. Such as they were, the concessions sounded too much like what they had been hearing from the health minister's officials during the previous, largely fruitless few months.

The meeting broke up with the junior doctors feeling frustrated, fobbed-off and angry. It seemed like the Howie campaign all over again. But the ministers walked out with a sense of accomplishment. They believed they had found a solution that recognised the junior doctors were overworked, but one that did not blow Bassett's budget. In short, in their mind a way out of the impasse had been achieved.

A few days later though, to the government's shock the junior doctors issued a statement warning of strike action. They had returned to the negotiating table, as they had promised at the meeting, but the talks had once again gone around in circles, only confirming the view of Cooper and his colleagues that the health ministry was determined to carry on as before and wear them out.

The ministers were furious at what they clearly saw as a snub. The usually equable Rodger fired off several terse telegrams to the Wellington office of the NZRMOA, warning them of the consequences. Bassett went public, describing talk of a strike as "irresponsible".

In the ensuing weeks pressure on the junior doctors mounted rapidly. It came from the hospitals, the government and even some of the junior doctors who were growing alarmed at where the campaign was heading. When they had signed up months earlier, few had thought it might come down to a full-scale strike. In the Wellington office the tension became too much for NZRMOA president Erihana Ryan who had connections with senior members of the government. In some distress she resigned her position and walked away from the campaign, in theory leaving the campaign without a titular leader. Her departure was not as much of a blow as it might have seemed because from the very start it had been the Auckland branch that had launched and carried the main burden, but it did weaken things at a crucial moment.

Back in his office in the government building universally dubbed "The Beehive" for its circular design, Bassett adopted a different tactic. He decided to outflank the campaign leaders by going over their heads and writing a letter to every junior doctor in the country outlining "the inconsistencies in their [representatives'] negotiating position." Encouraged by the response he got from some of them, the health minister became convinced the government had headed off any possibility of a strike. This view was confirmed to his satisfaction when, on September 7, the junior doctors resumed negotiations, albeit "with an ill grace", as the minister later noted.

Once again though, the negotiations dragged on without meaningful result and this time the junior doctors' patience was definitively exhausted. In all these months they had made almost no progress on the substantive issues laying on the table. After consulting with other ringleaders, they made a decision. If the only way they could achieve a result was by mounting a strike, then they would do so. They embarked on a nationwide tour of meetings with junior doctors in which they explained the situation and requested their support. Despite some reluctance, they got it.

And, taking a deep breath, they issued formal notice to the hospitals of strike warning. The nation's junior doctors would down tools on Sunday October 19, ten full months after the launch of the campaign.

Immediately, the prospect of a full-blown strike became the hot topic in hospital canteens all over New Zealand. The unthinkable had become a probability. "It was quite stressful even to think about it because it had never been done before," remembers neurologist Elizabeth Walker.

As the possibility of junior doctors walking out of the wards hit the headlines of a largely sympathetic media, the cartoonists enjoyed another field day, ten years after the Howie campaign. The Auckland Star's Bromhead sketched a burly hard-hatted worker from Marsden Point, an oil refinery project notorious for industrial stoppages, sitting in a chair before a bleary-eyed doctor slumped over his desk. Above the cartoon is the line: "House surgeons average earnings of $480 working a 100-hour week. Marsden Point workers average earnings of $976 working a 56-hour week." The doctor advises his patient: "You'll be glad to know that the lump on your backside isn't malignant. It's your wallet."

In the background Trott feared that things were getting out of hand. The last thing he wanted was a strike. As a young lawyer studying at the London School of Economics in the late 1970s, he had a ringside seat to the epic battles in the UK between militant unions and the government that became known as the Winter of Discontent. After returning to New Zealand and working for the Federation of Labour as an advocate, he had been drawn into other bitter disputes over strike action. And later, as a private negotiator Trott had been forced to extricate some of his clients from strikes that had run into dead-ends.

"All this very much coloured my view of the wisdom of *not* being caught in strike action with government forces," he recalls. "Strikes are easy to start but hard to end, and they often lead to messy results. Very quickly the dispute turns from issues of safe working conditions, for example, to the rule-of-law. Who runs the country?"

On the sidelines of the negotiations Trott had assiduously continued to cultivate members of the Higher Salaries Commission and other influential officials within government. "I was looking for a way out of the impasse as soon as it became clear that government ministers and their bureaucrats were not going to construct a settlement for the junior doctors," he says. "The negotiations were like ping-pong. I realised the ministers didn't want to touch this with a barge pole."

This was where the Higher Salaries Commission came into the picture. New Zealand's senior wage-fixing body, it was composed mainly of lawyers and accountants who had been appointed by Stan Rodger. The HSC had been established a decade earlier as a non-partisan organisation to fix the remuneration of the country's top officials including the prime minister, members of parliament, the judiciary and even the governor-general without the usual interference from politicians and other pressure groups interested in the outcome.

After informally sounding out the commission's views, Trott had to his considerable relief learned its members were open to at least a consideration of the junior doctors' claim. In fact, they seemed well-disposed to help in any way they could. "My strategy was to make the commission understand that they could get the government off the hook here," he recalls.

When negotiations collapsed for the last time, he decided the time was ripe to launch his own outflanking manoeuvre. "It's the only way to break the stalemate," he told his clients. "The commission can play the white knight." With his clients' agreement he duly filed the junior doctors' claim with the HSC. Like the initial document presented to the health ministry, it was carefully framed around the issue of overtime payments because Trott wanted to make it as easy as possible for the members to give a ruling. In doing so though, he had no illusions that the health officials – and probably the health minister -- would be put out by being side-lined. After all, having no idea that Trott had been cultivating the commission, they were completely in the dark.

With the claim filed, it was just a question of waiting to see what would happen.

Chapter seven

Bomb shell

As the clock ticked down to the day of the strike on October 19, emergency rosters were drawn up. Senior doctors in the nation's hospital had been alerted that they would be required to take over the junior doctors' duties in the acute wards. Others were put on notice they might be needed, depending on how long the strike lasted. Plans were made to admit only the more serious cases into A&E.

In the final week the junior doctors went about their normal duties, albeit increasingly nervous at the prospect of making history in a way they had never wanted or expected. But their nerve continued to hold and Cooper was confident the rebels had enough support for a general withdrawal of labour.

In Wellington the government was on the hook, caught between unleashing a torrent of budget-wrecking pay claims and keeping the hospitals running smoothly. It was too late to put an offer on the table because ministers had told the junior doctors in no uncertain terms that the government would not negotiate under the threat of a strike. Its only hope was that the rebels would crack and return to the wards, as junior doctors had done before.

The media widely deplored a situation that had been allowed to develop over most of the year and castigated the government for failing to act over such an important issue of public health.

The members of the Higher Services Commission had been studying the claim for weeks, still unknown to the government and health ministry. Trott, who remained on standby in Wellington, continued to keep his counsel while privately hoping a solution would be reached.

On Friday October 17, the last day that the commission could issue a determination before the strike, Trott made a snap decision to drop into the health ministry's buildings. He had an inkling that something was afoot. Just as he was about to enter, he bumped into one of the ministry's negotiators who was on the way out. The latter had received a surprise summons from the commission and was jumping into a taxi.

"I'll go with you," offered Trott. They shared the taxi in a state of considerable apprehension. The only difference was that the health ministry had no idea what this was all about while Trott was pretty sure he did.

The commission members did not waste any time. After a few preliminaries and handshakes, their decision was handed over and Trott and the ministry official withdrew to read it. Both were in a state of shock, albeit for different reasons. The commission had given the junior doctors practically everything they asked for – an increase of 15 per cent in basic pay plus hefty compensation for overtime. Almost as importantly, they were henceforth guaranteed a permanent place in their own right at the negotiating table instead of being lumped in with senior doctors. Even better, they would be automatically in line for an annual pay rise under a law called the State Services Conditions of Employment Act, a situation that was much more preferable from their viewpoint than having pay and conditions determined every three years by the Higher Salaries Commission, particularly at a time of high inflation.

In short the junior doctors had achieved a total victory while the ministry had been comprehensively outflanked.

As soon as he could excuse himself from the meeting, Trott rang Cooper who was working at the acute ward in Auckland Hospital. "You're not going to believe this," he announced. "We've won the whole lot. They've given us everything."

It was Cooper's turn to be stunned as he digested the news. After nearly a year of planning and negotiating under increasing tension as the stakes rose higher and higher, all the while fighting mounting exhaustion, the junior doctors had finally come through. Following decades of failures, their campaign to achieve decent and humane working conditions for junior doctors was successful. With the relief, he felt an overwhelming sense of achievement. As soon as got off the phone with Trott, he rang Swinburn who was working in another part of the hospital and broke the news. "Where are you now?" Cooper asked.

"In the gastro clinic."

"Right, I'm coming over." As soon as they met, they embraced and danced an impromptu victory jig in the hospital corridor to the amusement of hospital staff. From there Cooper went straight to the cafeteria where a group of colleagues were snatching something to eat between shifts. "We've won!" he announced.

The news was greeted with tired cheers – some of the junior doctors were finishing night-and-day shifts -- and exclamations of relief. They would not have to go on strike!

"At last we could stop hammering away and making threats," remembers Elizabeth Walker. "Finally, I could get on with my job and my career."

Back in the Beehive in Wellington, the mood could hardly have been more different. Fully comprehending the consequences, the government was appalled. They had been utterly blind-sided by a body – the Higher Salaries Commission -- whose very involvement in the matter came as a complete shock. Some ministers were furious, none more so than associate finance minister Prebble who could see coming an avalanche of hefty pay claims from the public sector. There was "no economic logic" whatsoever in the determination, he said.

It was crazy, he fulminated in the media, to set public-sector salaries according to relativities in the private sector, which was exactly what he considered the commission had done. And warming to his task, he criticised the whole idea of paying professionals overtime when they should, in his estimation, be remunerated for the quality of their work rather than the length of time they spent doing it. The long hours that junior doctors worked in hospitals were the logical outcome of their desire to learn. And drawing a long bow, he even attributed New Zealand's unimpressive rate of economic growth to the methodologies employed by the commission. (The minister must have forgotten it was those same methodologies that determined his own salary and other entitlements.)

Having lambasted the commission, the minister next turned his ire on the junior doctors, implying they were greedy and even lazy. There was "something obscene", he went on, when a 24 year-old could earn $60,000 a year while spending a significant amount of working time asleep. Clearly, the detailed survey of junior doctors' inordinately long shifts had not been drawn to his attention.

A genial if rumbustious personality, Prebble had a reputation for firing from the hip and he was clearly unaware that a whole ten years earlier the Howie campaign had won junior doctors the right to overtime payments. Nor could he have seen the Close Up documentary that followed Swinburn around the wards. If he had, it would surely have given him an insight into the punishing hours and relentless pressure that junior doctors had to bear on a daily basis.

The milder-mannered Bassett took a softer line, at least in public. Although the media described him as "privately concerned about the grave financial implications" of the ruling because it might trigger cuts in hospital services, he went on record to say the pay rises were generous and hoped they would make it easier to recruit junior doctors as a result. Behind the scenes though, he expressed his exasperation, complaining to his colleague and friend Stan Rodger that the junior doctors would now be paid while they slept. His main concern was that the ruling had blown the health budget sky-high. Ministry officials wasted no time in drawing up preliminary numbers that suggested the junior doctors would henceforth earn a 60 per cent increase for overtime on top of the 15 per cent hike in basic pay.

The government believed it had been outwitted and some Labour stalwarts remained resentful for years. After all, they had not been put in office by the medical profession, which historically supported the National party, and yet it was Labour that had ended up giving what the New Zealand Medical Journal gleefully described as a "doctors' bonanza."

As for the hospital boards, the fine print was dismaying. The determination made it crystal-clear that junior doctors – house surgeons and registrars – could no longer be rostered for the usual massive shifts without incurring hefty penalties in overtime payments. Nor could the new arrangements have come at a worse time for the hospitals because of the shortage of medical graduates, a problem that could be laid at the door of the previous government. As health department officials estimated, the hospitals faced an immediate shortfall of 55 doctors and, not far down the line, an extra 155 extra house surgeons would have to be found from somewhere.

The hospitals had roughly a year to put in place these radically new arrangements. But did they have a way out?

Even amid the euphoria of victory, Trott was concerned that the government might find a way to squash the commission's decision. This could be done on the basis that, because its implementation would trigger a queue of extravagant and economically ruinous wage claims, a responsible government could claim to be duty-bound to act in the national interest. "My principal concern was that the government would intervene on what was in effect a result of compulsory arbitration and legislate to overturn it," Trott remembers.

After all, it had happened before. Exactly six years earlier, the Federation of Labour had tried to resurrect a law called the General Wage Orders Act as a ploy to raise minimum hourly rates. Calling the federation's bluff, the autocratic Muldoon simply brushed the tactic aside with the simple expedient of making a television appearance to announce the act would be summarily repealed and taken off the statute books, leaving the federation high and dry. "And that's exactly what happened," notes Trott.

So, mindful of the potential consequences, Trott made sure to play down the terms of the settlement rather than rub salt in the government's wound. When contacted by the media seeking a victory statement, he adopted a measured tone. "We didn't get everything we wanted," he said judiciously. "It was a fair settlement".

The junior doctors took a similar line. Although delighted to have won the day, they could see that the implementation of the settlement would require upheavals in the hospital system and very likely trigger some antagonism at senior levels. So after the media had moved on to other stories, they kept their heads down, returned to work and dived into their studies.

In the passage of time Bassett recovered his usual equanimity and, in a review of a stormy year, seemed almost to believe the commission had done everybody a favour. Describing his department's achievements as "little short of spectacular," he noted that both senior and junior hospital doctors had enjoyed "a bonanza year" (echoing the New Zealand Medical Journal) and acknowledged that salaries had fallen badly behind. Two months later though, in a briefing to the Labour caucus the minister described the junior doctors' as having been "deluged with money". In the minister's opinion the medical profession in general owed a huge debt of gratitude to Labour. Quite apart from the money that had rained down on junior doctors, nurses salaries had jumped by between 28 and 48 per cent while those for full-time hospital specialists by an average of 36 percent. (Impressed by the success of their juniors' campaign, senior doctors had borrowed some of their ideas when they went into battle over their own salaries.)

Now that reform had been forced on the government, Bassett saw virtue in it. "The number of hours worked was reduced drastically for junior doctors", he enthused, which was to the great benefit of patients who would have the confidence the former were "not suffering from lack of sleep." Further, there would be an extra 160 junior doctors on the wards by early 1986, many of them hired from overseas with funds his officials had managed to scrape up from their heavily damaged health budget.

The intense publicity surrounding the junior doctors' campaign, with newspaper headlines running for months on end about the parlous state of the nation's hospitals, brought further unwanted consequences on Bassett's head. Shortly after the commission's bombshell, nearly all of Auckland's local bodies joined forces to slam the city's health services and demand a full-scale investigation by the health ministry. In a petition that contained the signatures of some of the most influential chairmen and mayors in the nation's biggest city, they sought an independent enquiry into the provision of psychiatric services, the distribution of accident and emergency services, and the general adequacy of hospital services in the poorer areas in the south and west.

This smacked of political grandstanding but, as if that wasn't enough, the complainants also wanted the enquiry to examine the conditions of employment for doctors and nurses in the wake of recurring allegations that patients had died because they had not received proper attention. Next, senior doctors began to clamour for an enquiry along the same lines. In Auckland, the hotbed of medical dissent, a ginger group of consultants gave a strong hint they were also prepared to stop work to discuss "the crisis in the public health system" as well as their own conditions of work.

The minister must have felt that, whatever he did, he could not win. Rather than taking it on the chin, he lashed out, rebuking local government leaders for blaming him for their own failures. Translated, it was up to the local authorities, not him, to run the hospitals properly.

The government's fears of inflationary knock-on settlements in the hospital sector were more than justified. Among other employees, laboratory staff and mortuary workers in Auckland went on strike in support of 30 per cent-plus wage claims. As the health minister would later note, "we stuffed their gobs with dollar notes."

The dam had burst.

Chapter eight

Aftermath

As soon as they had tied up the loose ends of the campaign, the ringleaders dived back into the hospital routine in the nick of time.

For months on end Cooper had been forced to skip the weekly lectures that all anaesthetic registrars were supposed to attend and his final specialist exams were looming. For the next eight months, he did little but work, sleep and study. In late 1986, he sat the exams, finishing top in Australasia, and spent the next year as a registrar in critical care before moving in 1987 to Seattle, a centre of excellence in anaesthesiology, to take up fellowship in trauma anaesthesia. He would stay there for the next four and a half years, thriving in a refreshingly different environment.

Swinburn, who had already passed his final exams, remained in New Zealand for a further two years. Succeeding Cooper, he assumed the presidency of the NZRMOA at a challenging time when the new working conditions were being bedded in. When his term was up, he also left for America, taking a post in the southwest of the USA where he would research the connection between diet, genetics and severe heart disease among other projects.

As for Mawson, after the drama of the campaign had died down he began to wonder if he and medicine were compatible. He enjoyed his extracurricular activities so much –SAS training, marathon running and hunting for *objets d'art* ("I haunted the antique shops and auction houses") – that he was uncertain whether medicine was his true vocation. "I wasn't sure I had made the right choice," he recalls. "Medicine wasn't a burning, all-consuming commitment for me." Indeed he even considered abandoning the profession in favour of opening an antique shop in London. Eventually though, he decided to persevere and complete his qualifications. Along the way though he discovered cardiac radiology, a specialty that enthralled him.

He also took a turn as president of the NZRMOA, succeeding Swinburn, and spent part of his time trying to explain to senior doctors what the campaign had really been about. That is, not money but working conditions. As he once reminded a meeting of the New Zealand division of Royal Australasian College of Surgeons, junior doctors' commitment and idealism had been exploited for far too long in a way that made the hospitals work better than would otherwise have been the case. "By maintaining standards and compensating for the inefficiencies and continual cost-cutting within the health service, we have protected the public from being made aware of the shambles that has developed over the last ten years," he said bluntly.

Mawson would also move abroad, in his case to Canada where he eventually settled. And he's been a specialist in cardiac radiology ever since.

After Elizabeth Walker put the campaign behind her, she was relieved to learn that her senior doctors did not file a negative report on her involvement. In due course she also left for the United States where she studied neurology at the Mayo Clinic before eventually returning to New Zealand.

In Dunedin, Paddy Dewan's involvement in the campaign and other causes, notably in training and patient care, caused friction between him and his bosses. Not a man to give up, he continued to argue for administrative reforms that would enable doctors to stay closer to their patients – he called it the "Patch Adams effect" after the movie starring Robin Williams. But he got little support and eventually this idealist went on to specialise in paediatric surgery in a career that would be marked by confrontation with senior management. Today he's heavily involved in humanitarian programmes such as Kind Cuts for Kids, an all-volunteer, Australia-based organisation that provides specialist medical care for children in developing countries. By 2017, Kind Cuts for Kids had treated over 3,000 children for life-threatening conditions.

Despite the initial fears of Cooper and his colleagues about how the HSC ruling would be implemented, the changes to junior doctors' conditions went through with surprising smoothness. In some regions the hospital boards dragged their feet and continued to roster junior doctors in much the same way as before, but generally the number of hours soon fell to the levels stipulated in the agreement.

It took time, goodwill and not a little ingenuity to develop the new rosters but problems were eventually resolved and the new shifts put in place. Shifts that comprised intensive, almost non-stop work where it was often impossible to grab a meal were capped at eight to ten hours. Continual work such as that undertaken by acute staff could be stretched to 16 hours. Intermittent work that offered some time off, such as in orthopaedics or general surgery when it might be quiet between midnight and dawn, could be rostered for 24 hours. And finally, the infrequent category of work – that is, light on-call duties – could be extended to three-day weekends or even for an entire week.

After the usual stormy incumbency in the health ministry, Bassett was removed by prime minister Lange after three and a half years, roughly the normal term for the job. His departure was no comfort to Bassett because he believed he was just getting to grips with a portfolio that he had enjoyed immensely, despite its manifest challenges. As he routinely pointed out, the public expects more from the health system than it can possibly deliver – "the sky is the limit to their expectations," he said in a prescient address a year before he lost office. Previous incumbents had said much the same thing.

And so did the members of the Higher Salaries Commission lose their jobs. Outraged that its members had issued a determination ahead of the hugely important wage round in the private sector in 1986, in effect sideswiping the government yet again without forewarning it, Stan Rodger refused to renew their warrants, as was his right. Neither he nor the government ever forgave the commission.

Following Bassett's departure, his own and succeeding governments continued to tinker with the hospital system, appointing various commissions that would investigate how to get more health bang for the buck. All of them ran into heavy opposition and heated debate before reforms were slowly achieved.

Once he had left public life, Bassett went on to become a distinguished political historian. More than 30 years later, he remains convinced the Labour government was ambushed by the junior doctors. "The big issue was always pay," Bassett says. "We were conned. As time went on, it became clear the real issue was pay."

Now a senior doctor in his old hospital, Cooper cordially denies this, reiterating what he had maintained all along during the campaign more than 30 years before. "I can honestly say we were always after better hours. We never believed that rules restricting hours would ever achieve this on their own. We knew that only the financial pressure of paying for overtime would create the incentive to reduce hours."

However in the years since he led the rebellion, there's no doubt that junior doctors in New Zealand have come to enjoy a privileged position in terms of salary largely because of the aggressive bargaining by their union, now called the Resident Doctors Association (RDA), that has long been run by another former junior doctor, Deborah Sidebotham. Over the years the RDA, which employs a full-time advocacy service, has had many a battle with the hospitals and government. Sidebotham hasn't hesitated to threaten or use strike tactics even when minor issues were involved, much to the irritation of senior staff including Cooper. Indeed so successful has agitation by the RDA been that junior doctors have somehow won the right to free meals during shifts, alone among hospital staff.

While they were furthering their experience in North America, Cooper and his colleagues had an unexpected ringside seat to one of the turning points there in the long-running saga over residents' conditions.

The Libby Zion affair had simmered away for two years before returning to the headlines because of a grand jury investigation that raised most of the New Zealand issues all over again, albeit on a much wider stage. Essentially, the grand jury's report found serious fault with the way the Zions' daughter had been treated at New York Hospital. From the moment of entry to the hospital, she had been seen only by residents who were in the early stages of training. Moreover the residents had been on their feet for 18 hours. Serious mistakes, the grand jury concluded, had been made in her medication and general treatment.

The clear implication from the findings was that Libby Zion could – and perhaps should -- have survived.

In the middle of a groundswell of protest about the allegedly deteriorating quality of hospital treatment, the release of the report triggered a full-scale enquiry into the state of emergency services in New York hospitals. Its chairman was Dr Bertrand Bell, the very man who had highlighted these issues years before. Among the enquiry's preliminary recommendations was one limiting shifts in emergency services to twelve hours -- pretty much what the New Zealand campaign had fought for -- and sixteen hours in non-emergency, plus a minimum eight-hour break in between. Another recommendation was for senior attending physicians to be present at certain crucial times in treatment.

In short it wasn't fair or appropriate to leave seriously ill patients in the hands of exhausted trainee doctors.

The economic implications of these recommendations were tremendous. As a detailed analysis by the Greater New York Hospital Association estimated, they would require the appointment of 2,045 specialists and 975 full-time equivalent ancillary personnel in 50 New York hospitals. The financial cost would be nearly $204 million per year.

In time these recommendations would be modified to meet economic considerations, but the Libby Zion case served to throw a spotlight on how residents were expected to work in America. For months on end the New England Journal of Medicine ran hot with impressively researched articles and letters, including one co-authored by Cooper and Swinburn that outlined what they had achieved in New Zealand two years earlier.

At his new post in Seattle Cooper had been shocked by some of the accepted practices. So restrictive were they that one neurosurgical chief resident, for example, was only able to see his children when they visited him in the canteen. If he was lucky, that might happen just once a week during an entire six-month shift when he was confined to the hospital. Cooper had also heard stories about residents in post-cardiac intensive care units in Texas hospitals who were required to stay on the ward for weeks at a time. One supposedly got into trouble for going down to the hospital car park to snatch a moment with his wife.

Invited to have his say by the New York attorney general's office, Swinburn made an appearance at the grand jury hearing in New York over the Libby Zion case. Much of the proceedings had been taken up by senior doctors who argued that endless hours were essential in training – but Swinburn presented an alternative view. He told the hearing how New Zealand had solved the very problem its members were wrestling with and, summarising the arguments, he put it neatly: "The world doesn't end just because junior doctors get some sleep."

Between them, the campaign leaders ended up briefing high-profile hearings in Boston, Seattle and Montreal. They also had the pleasure of meeting Libby Zion's father who was more than interested in the changes that had been brought about in New Zealand. Everywhere they went, the arguments against reform were much the same as they had encountered back home. First, long training hours were supposedly essential to the creation of good doctors. Second, the design of rosters that allow residents to get some sleep would mean the hiring of more doctors. Third, extra doctors would cost money. And fourth, if this went on, there would soon be a surplus of doctors.

One of their most attentive audiences was the National Federation of House Staff Organisations, a body of interns similar but much larger than the NZRMOA, at a conference in Boston in early 1988. The message they gave must have been music to the interns' ears. It had not proved impossible, as the pessimists had predicted, to come up with a workable roster. "Contrary to the belief before the system changed, the actual number of rosters that were difficult to draw up and implement were surprisingly few, a very small minority," explained Mawson.

He went on to say the biggest reform was probably in the issue of handovers, albeit after some teething problems. "There needs to be one or in some cases two hours overlap in people arriving and people leaving the hospital so that proper handovers can be conducted," he concluded.

For Swinburn one of the biggest improvements was in training — the primacy of quality over quantity. "Quantity quickly becomes counter-productive when fatigue sets in. Residents who are sleep-deprived switch to automatic pilot," he said. The heads of his audience would surely have nodded in agreement.

In fact the bad old days of "mileage" were already on the way out. The more forward-looking medical colleges were turning to skill-based assessments, simulation training, log books for certain types of cases and other more enlightened methods of teaching.

But perhaps most importantly, the reforms had ushered in a more pleasant as well as productive hospital environment. As Cooper put it: "No patient should ever be treated by a sleep-deprived doctor. Patients in need of care at 4am now expect to see an awake, alert, interested and very tolerant doctor. Productivity at night has increased. Nurses find the doctors easier to deal with. At a personal level, if I was rostered to start work at 8pm under the new regulations, I arrive ready for the job, really happy to work as an intensive care registrar."

And surely it was a bonus, he added, that junior doctors now had more time with their families and leisure to pursue outside interests. "Enthusiasm for one's job is high," Cooper told the American residents. "Excessive tiredness should be a thing of the past."

Looking back, it's hard to fathom how extreme fatigue was ever thought to be a prerequisite in the provision of sometimes life-saving medicine.